SURVIVING ALZHEIMER'S

Martha L. Johnson

MARTHA L. JOHNSON

SURVIVING ALZHEIMER'S

A Caregiver's Story

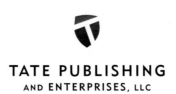

TATE PUBLISHING
AND ENTERPRISES, LLC

Published by Tate Publishing & Enterprises, LLC
127 E. Trade Center Terrace | Mustang, Oklahoma 73064 USA
1.888.361.9473 | www.tatepublishing.com

Tate Publishing is committed to excellence in the publishing industry. The company reflects the philosophy established by the founders, based on Psalm 68:11,
"The Lord gave the word and great was the company of those who published it."

Book design copyright © 2014 by Tate Publishing, LLC. All rights reserved.
Cover design by Rhezette Fiel
Interior design by Honeylette Pino

Published in the United States of America

ISBN: 978-1-62854-196-0
1. Medical / Geriatrics
2. Medical / Mental Health
13.11.22

DEDICATION

In honor of my Heavenly Father for all of His love that He gives to each and every one of His children. Also this is in memory of my father-in-law, Richard E. Johnson, who suffered from the disease of Alzheimer's for fifteen years.

To all of the members of Hagood Avenue Baptist Church in Barnwell, South Carolina, and their families who knew how to show love and kindness to those that are suffering from Alzheimer's disease.

ACKNOWLEDGMENTS

Most of all I want to thank God for being the main reason that I am writing this book. God gave Roger and I the dream to help families in this world know what Alzheimer's disease can do to their families. I also want to thank Him for carrying me in His arms and loving me when I was in the most difficult time in my life. Thank you, God, for loving each and every one of your children.

I want to praise my Lord for having given me my best friend—someone who knew just when I needed to be loved, encouraged, and supported. And when times were hard and the road of life was difficult, I didn't have to travel it alone. I would like to take this time to thank my loving husband, Roger, for keeping me on the path that God has in store for me with this book.

I want to thank Matthew, Benjamin, Miranda, Emory, and Everett for being a part of my life and for encouraging me to do God's work. Also for helping me out with their grandfather when I needed their help. Emory and Everett, you both are a gift from God, and we love you so very much. You came into our lives at the most difficult time, but you brought peace with your little smile that lights up the whole world.

God sent me another family when I needed one to care for me while my world was falling apart around me. They showed me what love and kindness are and how to answer the call of God—that is, to care for each other. If it was not for each and every members of Hagood Avenue Baptist Church, I don't know what I would have done by myself.

> Jesus asks Simon Peter do you truly love Me? Peter answered yes, Jesus told Peter to care for His sheep. God ask of each of us that same question, and as a church you answered yes.
>
> John 21:16 (NIV)

I have asked our Lord to keep you all in His care and that you remember that you will always be my family. Thank you for loving me always.

Most of all I would like to thank Dr. Patricia Parmelee, Ph.D., director of the Center for Mental Health and Aging and Department of Psychology, at the University of Alabama; Cheryl Thrasher, ALA, executive director of Lakeview Estates; and Connie Rockett, RN; MSN educator for several company throughout the State of Alabama, for all their help with my research and teaching me more about Alzheimer's/dementia disease. Most of all, thank you for being on the REJAF foundation board of directors. May God keep you all in his care and love always. Thank you for all your help.

I would like to thank all the staffs at Ashton Gables, Covered Bridge, and Hampton Oaks for the love and care that you showed to each one of your residences and their families.

Thank you to the Johnson family for inspiring this book and in letting our family story be told. I pray that our story will help other families that have a loved one suffering with Alzheimer's disease.

If it was not for the helpful information that the Alzheimer's Foundation of America, Alzheimer's Association, and the Mayo Clinic has given me, I would not have been able to care for my father-in-law in such a loving and caring way.

I also would love to thank the staff of Tate Publishing for helping me see that *Surviving Alzheimer's: A Caregiver's Story* finds its way into the hands of our readers.

I hope this book will bring some comfort to the families that have or will have a loved one that has been diagnosed with Alzheimer's disease.

CONTENTS

Personal Christian Beliefs Statement......................15

Foreword...17

Introduction...19

Our Family Story About How Alzheimer's
disease Came Into Our Lives..............................25

What Is Alzheimer's?.....................................29

Warning Signs 31

Diagnosis..37

Seven Diseases That Attack the Mind 39

    Huntington's Disease 39

    Parkinson's Disease 45

    Wilson's Disease 50

    Vascular Dementia 53

    Lewy Body Dementia 55

    Frontotemporal Dementia 57

    Posterior Cortical Atrophy (PCA) 60

Symptoms...67

Life Expectancy 75

Treatment 77

Statistics 79

Cost 81

Caregivers Get Sick Themselves 83

Tips for Caregivers 85

    Putting Together a Daily Routine for a
    Person with Alzheimer's.........................90

    Caregivers Need to Have Some Personal Time......93

How to Look for a Good In-Home
 Caregiver's Services..95
Tips for the Holidays..97
Communication..107
Daily Actives 113
 Art 113
 Music..116
 Storytelling 118
Pictures..121
Projects You Can Make with or for Your Loved
 Ones 125
 Care Box..125
 Memory Book..127
 Music Album 128
 Story Board..128
Making Your Home Safe for Your Loved One 131
Asking Your Doctor Questions about
 Alzheimer's Disease 135
 These Are Some of the Important Things
  That You Need to Do and Take
  to the Doctor Appointments........................135
 Emergency Room Visits 136
Lifestyle Choices 139
 Stress Management..141
Prescription Drug Coverage 145
Educational Resources..147
 State Government Resources (Alabama)..........147
 Federal Government Resources........................147
Long-Term Care..151
 Making It Easier for Our Loved One to
  Transition to Residential Care Settings 158

How to Plan for Long-Term Care 164
Paying for Long-Term Care............................. 175
Legal and Financial Planning............................. 185
The Conclusion... 191
Notes 193

PERSONAL CHRISTIAN BELIEFS STATEMENT

In the beginning from the time that Roger and I first accepted Jesus Christ as our Lord and Savior, we knew that even though we were a Christians, our lives would have lots of bumps and bruises along the way. We believe that the gospel is God's Holy Word and that God the Father, God the Son, and God the Holy Spirit are one.

In 1982 I moved to Dallas, Texas, to work for one of the world's top slack company, as their assistant designer in women's wear. While working there, one of my coworkers asked me if I would like to attend church with her. It was there where I met Roger, and on February 23, 1985, we were married. In 1987 we started our family with the birth of our first son, Matthew, and in 1989 our second son, Benjamin, came into the world.

Roger's career has taken us from Dallas, Texas; to Logan, Utah; Anderson, South Carolina; and to Barnwell, South Carolina. In 2006, we had to move Roger's parents in with us because Roger's dad had been diagnose with Alzheimer's disease, and his mom needed to have more help with his father's care.

In 2007, I was left with the care of Roger's parents, while he began working for Century Tube in Madison, Indiana. I feel this is where God carried me in His arms, and this is also when my faith grew. I trusted that what I was going through would help me in my walk with God. It would be through my time spent with Him that I would gain the strength to go on caring for my father- and mother-in-law. I leaned heavily on what God tells us that "He is our refuge and strength even in time of trouble" (Psalm 46:1, NIV).

As I was having my difficulties back in South Carolina, in Indiana, Roger was feeling helpless that he could not help me with everyone and everything back home. He rested in the fact that I had already given this matter to the Lord. I needed him to do his job in Indiana, but like a good husband, he still felt helpless in caring for his family. God tells us that we need to "trust in the Lord with all our heart and He will take care of us in our time of need" (Proverbs 3:5, NIV)

I believe that in having faith in God and walking with Him daily, we come to know how wonderful a Father he is, how much he loves His children and wants them to come to know Him. "That who ever received and believed in the Father will be given the right to become children of God" (John 1:12, NIV).

FOREWORD

Who is affected by the person with Dementia? This book will show how one person can touch and change the lives of many people. So the answer to that question is that one person with Dementia touches everyone they come in contact with and everyone can make a change. 5.4 million Persons are suffering with the disease of Alzheimer's. This means that one out of eight persons will be diagnosed at a rate of every 68 seconds with this disease. It is projected that Alzheimer's will quadruple in the next 50 years and is now the 6th leading cause of death in the United States with a 66% of Alzheimer deaths in the US. With these statistics, it is a great possibility that you will have someone in your life that will be diagnosed with Alzheimer's or it could be you that is the one out of the eight.

There are over 15,000,000 caregivers in the U.S. If there was one state made up of all these caregivers, it would be the 5th largest state in the United States. Being a caregiver will challenge your emotions and physical abilities. It causes fatigue and sometimes the feeling of isolation.

Surviving Alzheimer: A Caregivers Story contains true stories from the personal experiences of a daughter-in-law caring for her father-in-law. These stories will allow you to feel the emotions through the eyes of the author. It will help prepare you to understand your loved ones changes along with assisting you in how to seek different types of support. It will give you information related to the disease process and ideas how to cope with the new and unexpected challenges. Alzheimer's brings unique behaviors and knowing these behaviors will help you with your communication and approach with the affected person. The more knowledge the caregiver has about the person's disease, the more support and realistic expectations they will have with assisting their loved ones through the Dementia Journey!

This book is to help you understand that is still your special love, who has a disease. The behaviors are the disease, not the person. These special persons deserve the best care and the best quality of life. As a caregiver it is exhausting but with hard work and love, it can bring you peace, memories and many achieving rewards.

Caregiver wanted! Requirements are having stamina, problems solving abilities and resiliency!

Be Prepared!

—Connie Rockett RN MSN

INTRODUCTION

My dear readers,

As a daughter-in-law who became a full-time caregiver and care manager to her father-in-law who had been diagnosed with Alzheimer's disease in 2002, I needed to find out all that I could about this disease. I wanted to give him the best care when he came to live with us in 2006.

Surviving Alzheimer's: A Caregiver's Story will contain a personal Christian belief statement. This faith statement will let the reader know that Christians too experience lots of bumps and bruises along the way. But it would be God who would guide and help us through this time in our lives, as we dealt with the disease of Alzheimer's.

The dedication page will show how much God loves us and knows just what we can handle. There will also be a church family that stepped in and did what God asked them to do. But mostly there will be a loving father-in-law that has the disease of Alzheimer's, which would slowly take away his memories.

The acknowledgments page will reveal many people and their love and help that played a very big part in *Surviving Alzheimer's: A Caregiver's Story*. Without their love and help, this book would not have come about.

The introduction will show my readers why the author has written *Surviving Alzheimer's: A Caregiver's Story*. She will also share her goals with her readers: on how Alzheimer's came to be a part of her family, how her family handled the warning signs, and the diagnosis of this disease. At the same time, she will educate her readers on the medical knowledge that is required to deal with this disease and more on her family story as it unfolds though out the book.

The author will take her readers on a journey through what Alzheimer's is, what the warning signs are, and how doctors diagnose this disease. She will introduce the top seven dementia and how they attack different sections of the brain. Martha will also help her readers to have a better understanding of what this disease can do to a person's memory.

At the same time, her readers will find out how symptoms, life expectancy, treatment, statistics, and cost come into play with the disease of Alzheimer's. This information will help families to prepare for this disease before it strikes a member of their family. As she continues to take her readers on this journey, she will bring them to a very importation part of this book called "Tips for the Caregiver." Here her readers will find helpful hints on ways to care for their loved ones. At the same time Martha will show her readers how to put together a daily routine that they and their loved one can follow, and as caregivers how to have some time off. When the time comes for the caregiver to need more help, *Surviving Alzheimer's: A Caregiver's Story* will help assist them on how to find good in home care service, as well on how to make the holidays fun and less stressful on both the caregiver and their loved one.

Thought *Surviving Alzheimer's: A Caregiver's Story* the author will teach her readers how very important it is to communicate in the right way with their loved one. For example, when using the five S's (simple, slow, show, smile, and speak) as caregivers we will be able to help our loved one be at ease when they are communicating with their family or friends. Communication can also be used through three types of therapy: art, music, and storytelling. Also along with communication and therapy methods, memory projects can be very useful to the family and can be very helpful to the nursing home or assisted-living facility, as the memory projects will give the nursing home or assisted-living facility a better look into their residences life. For example, a care box plays a big role in the way that families care for their loved ones when they have to take their loved one to the doctor, hospital, or on and outing.

Memory books, music memory books, and story boards are good ways for children to learn more about their grandparents. It is also a good way to bring learning and fun together for the whole family.

As Martha continues to take her readers on the journey though *Surviving Alzheimer's: A Caregiver's Story*, they will learn how to safe-proof their homes to reduce accidents and increase their loved ones' well-being as their loved one lives with the disease of Alzheimer's. Safe-proofing your home will give you (the caregiver) peace of mind and will reduce your stress level.

One of the most important things that a caregiver need to do is to keep asking the doctor questions about

Alzheimer's disease. As well as keep up with all the important paperwork that needs to be taken to the doctor's or emergency room.

When going to the emergency room, see that the physicians know that your loved one has Alzheimer's disease and what stage your loved one is in. Stay with your loved one, answer all the doctors' questions, make sure that you have brought all the paperwork that will be needed in the emergency room; this should include your Power of Attorney (POA) for health, a copy of do-not-resuscitate orders, living will, medications, ID, insurance cards, key people to call, and their numbers. Don't forget the care box, memory book, or the music album. This will be good for your loved one's stress level, while they wait for the doctor. Ask if there is another room or a quiet place where you can wait. A person with Alzheimer's disease does not like noise, bright lights, or crowds. Putting your loved one into this type of environment will increase stress and agitation.

Martha will also help her readers to care for their brain health, have a more rewarding lifestyle, and how to manage their stress level. At the same time she will give her reader's very important information on prescription drug coverage, educational resources, and she will also guide her readers's on how to plan, pay, and find the right long-term care; as well as help their loved one transition into resident care. Martha will also tell her readers about the most important matters that need to be taken care of immediately before her readers loved one becomes incapacitated, and that is to see that all their legal and financial matters are put in order.

In the conclusion, Martha will bring her reader to the end of her story, it would be her hope that her reader will have a better understanding of what Alzheimer's is, how this disease will affect their family and most of all how very important it is to have Jesus Christ in our lives, for families to be able to survive Alzheimer's disease. We all need to remember that family and friends go home at the end of the day. But God will never leave His children in their time of need.

OUR FAMILY STORY ABOUT HOW ALZHEIMER'S DISEASE CAME INTO OUR LIVES

I would like to tell you a story about how Alzheimer's came to be a part of our family. In December 2002, our family went to Austin, Texas, to celebrate my husband's parents'(Richard and Nancy Johnson, though out the book Richard and Nancy will be call Dad and Mom. In our family this is how we refer to our parents. We don't refer to our parent as in-law, to us this show disrespect to our elder.) fiftieth wedding anniversary. We were surprising Mom (Nancy) and Dad (Richard) that all three of their children (Roger, Craig, and Camille) and their families had come home for their anniversary and Christmas.

When we walked into the house, Dad did not recognize his sons (Roger, and Craig) for several minutes. At dinner that night, I could see that he was having a hard time keeping up with the conversation at the table. He even had a hard time ordering his dinner. I kept watching him and could see that he was doing a lot of repeating of sentences and stories that night. I bent over to my husband and told him that something was wrong with his dad.

That night when we all got back to our hotel, we began to talk about what we had seen. Roger and his brother decided they needed to have a talk with their sister to see if she could convince Mom to make an appointment for Dad to see the doctor and find out what was wrong with him.

The very next week, Camille asked her mother to make an appointment for Dad. Mom said their father did not need to see the doctor; he was fine.

With Alzheimer's/Dementia, denial is very common in all members of the family. Each member will react in different ways towards the possibility of a loved one having the disease of Alzheimer's.

One night about two weeks after we came back from Texas, Camille called and told us that she was having a hard time getting Mom to make an appointment for Dad. After some time, Mom came to her senses, and she finally made the appointment.

On the day of the appointment, we called to find out what had happened at the doctor's. Mom told Roger what the doctor had said. The results from the test confirmed our suspicions that Dad did have Alzheimer's. Now Roger and I had to talk about how we were going to care for his parents.

In December 2005, Roger and his brother went to Texas to have a talk with their parents, to see if they would move to South Carolina where we could see to their care and needs. At the end of February, Roger and Craig returned to Texas to get Dad and Mom ready to move to South Carolina. It would be through this time that I would start to do research on the disease to find out what Alzheimer's was. This was my first step in dealing with the disease. My life was about to change, not only was I going to be taking care of my family. Now I would become a full time caregiver to Dad and Mom.

You might be asking yourself why a Daughter-in-Law's would be caring for her husband parents. Well the following reason was that my husband had to move to Madison, Indiana for his job, as for my brother-in-law (Craig) he would pass away in February 2007, my sister-in-law (Camille) lives in Texas and traveling was very costly for her, to be able to come once a month. So you can see that I was the only one that was left to see to Dad and Mom care, and the other reason was that our Lord also called me to do a job, and show the world that caring for parents is not just a one sided family job. It's alright for Daughters or Sons-in-law to care for their father and mother-in-law just as they can care for their parents as well.

Not only will I tell you my story, but I will also teach you what the disease of Alzheimer's will do to your loved ones memory. In the next chapter we will define what Alzheimer's disease is.

WHAT IS ALZHEIMER'S?

What is Alzheimer's? Alzheimer's is a disease that attacks the nerve cells of the brain. As a caregiver that had a father-in-law with Alzheimer's disease. I have seen firsthand, how Alzheimer's come into a person life. Alzheimer's didn't attack Dad brain all at once; it comes on little by little over our time. As time went on we (Family) could see how Alzheimer's disease was inhibits his ability to thinking, used language skills and we could see how Dad behavior was changes as the disease advance in his life.

By now you are asking yourself what causes the disease we call Alzheimer's. Researchers state that Alzheimer's is when plaque and neurofibrillary tangles take over the brain.

1. *"Beta-amyloid plaque.* A sticky clump of protein fragments and cellular material that form outside and around neurons. (The nerve cells of the brain)
2. *Neurofibrillary tangles.* Insoluble twisted fiber composed largely of the protein tau that builds up inside the nerve cells."[1]

Researchers are unclear that plaque and neurofibrillary tangles are the main cause of Alzheimer's. "The Alzheimer's Education and Referral Centers are now telling us that Alzheimer's may be caused by many factors, like the following,

1. Age is identified as the highest risk factor of this disease.
2. Genetic makeup is made up by what is passed down through our families.
3. Oxidative damage to nerve cell from the overproduction of toxic free radicals—like smoking, alcohol, or drug abuse.
4. Serious head injuries.
5. Brain inflammation.
6. Environmental factors."[2]

Alzheimer's is not a psychological disease, but it is more a medical condition that attacks our brain cells.

In the next chapter we will look at the warning signs that will help us as caregivers to understand what is happening to our loved ones memory. Here I will add my story so you can have a better understanding of what went on with Dad as his family started to see the warning signs appear in him.

WARNING SIGNS

Like all diseases, warning signs let us know that we have a problem that needs to be taken care of. The first step we need to take is to see that our loved ones see the doctor right away. The doctor will be able to find out what the problem is, how to fix the problem, or if we need to see a specialist.

Let's look at how memory loss can affect our lives.

I would like to take you through the next part of our story dealing with the disease of Alzheimer's and how I came to see the warning signs in Dad after he came to live with us in South Carolina.

Thinking. By the time Dad came to South Carolina he had already lost the ability to use his mind to reason, form thoughts, make judgments, and to come up with ideas.

Language skills. As for using language, Dad didn't like to talk to people. Here is an example that will help you to have a better understanding.

As for speaking, Dad did very little; (when I say very little I mean a nod of the head or a smile) he would only talk to people that he knew or members of his family that he would see daily. When my brother-in-law and his wife would come once in a while, to give us a break, Dad would not speak to them very much. I would have to explain to them that Dad was having a hard time communicating with people that he doesn't see every day.

See, a person with Alzheimer's disease has a very hard time remembering who people are when they don't see them for a long period of time.

Behavior change. Dad's behavioral changes played a big part in how he dealt with life with Alzheimer's disease.

When it came to Dad's behavior, I could see lots of changes taking place. This is an example of how I handled his behavior when it would get out of hand. He was a man that was assertive when he did not have Alzheimer's. As a person with the disease, he became more passive and emotional. When something would happen to him or Mom, he would get very angry, and his temper would flare up. (These are just a few situations that affected his behavior. Getting dressed, taking a bath, he would get mad because you asked him to do something that he didn't want to do or you had to get him up from a nap early to go to the doctor would get his behavior off to a bad start.)

The first thing I would do was to calm myself down and ask God to help me through this problem with Dad. This made it easier for me to calm Dad down and find out what made him so angry.

Then I would take Mom into another room and have a talk with her, to let her know that when Dad gets angry, he does not understand why he is angry, and his anger could lead him to hit someone. The reason that I would have a talk with Mom was about two months after they moved to South Carolina and into their own home. One day when I was unpacking their things, Mom ask Dad to come and take a bath. He told her, "No," and she would try to explain to him that he had not had a bath in a week, and he needed to take one. I heard her voice go up several octaves, and I ran to see what was going on. Dad had Mom by the wrist and she was trying to tell him to let go. I step in and told Dad let go of Mom you are hurting her or I will call the Sheriff. That did the trick, and from that moment on I always had a talk with Mom when Dad got very mad at every one. At the same time, I knew that Mom was still in denial over her husband having Alzheimer's. She did not understand that he now needed her help. (See Mom was use to Dad taking care of her, and it was hard for her to put her husband needs before hers, she was sick herself with heart disease as well as chronic obstructive pulmonary disease (COPD). "God tells us that He made man and woman to be helpers to each other" (Genesis 2:18, NIV); With Alzheimer's/ dementia, denial is very common in all members of the family. Each member will react in different ways toward the possibility of a loved one having the disease of Alzheimer's.

Now this meant that it was up to me to see to Dad's care as well as Moms.

Not remembering where they placed objects. One of the first warning signs we (family) will see in our loved one, will be where they have place objects. For example, when I would go over to Dad and Mom's house (Dad and Mom were live on their own for about one year after they moved to South Carolina. Mom had a heart attack and my husband was getting ready to move out of state, and Mom heart doctor didn't want them to be on

their own anymore. So we moved them into our home.)
to see how they were doing, on a daily basis, Dad was
always looking for something. I would ask him, "What
are you looking for, Dad?" He would tell me that he was
looking for his house keys, eyeglasses, even his shoes,
or other things that he did not remember where he
had placed them. He would laugh when I would find
whatever he was looking for. One of the things that I
first noted was cups of coffee all over the house, when
they lived on their own.

Not recognizing the names and faces of people. Dad
even had a hard time recognizing his two sons Roger
and Craig, daughter Camille, and as well as his six
grandchildren for some time in the beginning stages of
his Alzheimer's. When Dad forgot his children, he still
could remember who his wife (Nancy) was in the early
stages, but as the Alzheimer's advanced, he began to
forget her as well. This made it very difficult for Mom
to deal with. They had been married for over fifty years,
and Mom never thought this was going to be the way it
was going to end, that her husband would live the rest
of his life not knowing who she was.

Important information. Like all family when you
bring your parents to live with you, there is a reason
why they can no longer live on their own. This example
will give you an idea why we had to move Dad and
Mom to South Carolina. Dad and Mom came to South
Carolina because they had made a bad decision with
their investments. A misleading salesman convinced
them to take their investment from their old company
and place them with his company. At the same time, he

told Dad and Mom that they could make more money with his company on their investments per year.

When my husband (Roger) found out what they had done, and they had not consulted him about this matter, he hit the roof. (Roger has a master's degree in finance.) They lost $12,000 in penalties by moving their investments. Shortly after Roger had been told about this matter, he returned to Texas with his brother (Craig) to have a heart-to-heart talk with their parents and to convince them to move to South Carolina. It would make it much easier for us to keep a close eye on their financial, legal, and medical affairs. This is why I am saying that we (caregivers or families) need to watch over our loved ones at all times.

When Dad and Mom came to South Carolina to live with us, the first thing I did was to get them in touch with an attorney. (Who knew elder law.) We wanted to make sure that all of their important papers were taken care of and to see that they named Roger as their Power of Attorney (POA) for financial, legal, and medical. Dad and Mom had also named me their POA for health only. I was going to be taking them to see their doctors most of the time. This was also recommended by their attorney. When we returned home from meeting with the attorney, I took all of the important papers out of Mom's desk and brought them home with us. I even started to pay all of their bills at the same time. This made life much easier for Roger and me.

Recent events. Recent events that took place in our family; for example, when Craig passed away in

February 2007, Roger took both of his parents to see the body before the funeral. Craig's wife was having his body cremated. Dad and Mom only had twenty-four hours to see the body, before they did the cremation. Dad did not understand who the person was. Roger had to tell his father that his son Craig had passed away. It was then that he could remember who Craig was, and he began to cry. Within minutes, he forgot why he was there. This broke Mom's heart that Dad could no longer remember that he had lost his son. (to cancer)

Please keep in mind that your loved one will have a very hard time with recent events that happen in your family. We made the decision to take Dad to the funeral with our hearts instead of looking at how this event would affect him. He did not like how people looked at him, and he could not even understand why they were telling him that they were sorry for his loss. What made it harder on the family was that people didn't understand that Dad was my brother-in-law's father, and he had the right to be at his son's funeral. We should not be ashamed when a family member has Alzheimer's. They are much a part of our family as we are.

Now the next chapter is going to help us to understand how doctors diagnosis the disease of Alzheimer's as well as other dementia diseases.

DIAGNOSIS

"Clinicians (Doctors) can now diagnose Alzheimer's disease within ninety percent accuracy, but one of the best ways that Alzheimer's can be confirmed is by an autopsy."[3] When I took Dad to see the doctor's for the first time, the doctor ask me question about our complete family medical history, and he then order lab tests, brain scans, and neuropsychological tests as well as a full physical exam. In the physical exam the doctor wanted to see if Dad was able to make judgment, pay attention, use language skills, and solve problems. "Alzheimer's can only be confirmed by an autopsy, during which pathologists look for the disease's characteristic plaques and tangles in brain tissue"[4]

A proper diagnosis is very important to a person with Alzheimer's. In today world there are many other causes of memory loss that can affect our lives. Memory loss can come though vitamin deficiencies, thyroid and depression. But doctor can help us by treat these problems. But there are other memory conditions that are not so easy to treat. In the next chapter we will take a closer look at these memory conditions.

SEVEN DISEASES THAT ATTACK THE MIND

There are about ninety different diseases and dementias that are attacking us, and new ones are being found every day. These are just a few to look at our brain today

HUNTINGTON'S DISEASE

Definition

"Huntington's disease is a disease that progresses over time; it causes the central nerve cells of our brain to waste away. As an outcome of this disease, a person can experience uncontrollable movements, emotional turmoil, and mental deterioration.

Huntington's disease is inherited from one generation to the next. Symptoms of Huntington usually develop around the age of 30s and 40s, and the disease progression may occur faster in a younger person.

There are medications that are available to help manage the symptoms of this disease, but treatments can't stop Huntington's from the physical and mental diminishment that this disease will do to the human brain." [5]

Symptoms

"Huntington's disease can vary from person to person. This disease usually develops slowly over time, and the severities of the symptoms are related to the level of loss in the nerve cell. Death occurs about ten to thirty years after the symptoms first appeared.

The early symptoms of Huntington's disease include the following:

A. Personality changes
   1. Irritability
   2. Anger
   3. Depression
   4. Lose interest in life
B. Reducing the thinking and reasoning abilities
   1. Making decisions
   2. Remembering new information and learning new skills
   3. Being able to answer questions
   4. Remember important information
C. Mild balance problems
D. Clumsiness
E. Involuntary facial movements such as grimacing

Family and friends may see these symptoms before we are aware that these symptoms are happening to us.

Huntington's disease also has symptoms that take place as the disease advances:

A. A sudden twitch
B. Severe problems with their balance and coordination
C. The twitch of rapid eye movements
D. Hesitant
E. Swallowing problems
F. Dementia
G. Seizures

If you have a history of Huntington's disease in your family and start to see these symptoms, please see your doctor right away." [6]

Causes

"The cause of Huntington's disease is a single abnormal gene that is inherited from either parents. It only takes one copy of the abnormal gene for a person to inherit Huntington's disease. If one parent has the abnormal gene their children have a 50 percent chance of inheriting the disease. Because the signs and symptoms don't appear until a person is in their mid 30s or 40s, parents may not know that they are carriers of this gene until they have children.

If a child does not inherit the abnormal gene, they will not have Huntington's disease and can't pass the gene on to the next generation. If the child does get the abnormal gene and within time they will show symptoms of this disease and can also pass the gene on to their children.

In 2006, researchers discovered that protein that is expressed by the Huntington's gene interacts with another protein to disturb the way that cholesterol is collected in the brain. Cholesterol is necessary for healthy brain cells, and the network among the brain cells needs the cholesterol to be in the correct levels and in the correct locations. When the network of the brain cells is destroyed, motor skills, thinking skills and speech will be affected. If scientists can find away to see that the interaction between the proteins and Huntington's gene can be disturbed in a way that cholesterol is collected in the correct way, then they may finally be able to develop a drug that can help Huntington's disease." [7]

Complications

"After the disease begins the symptoms will continue until death. Even though the symptoms will be different from person to person, vital functions, as swallowing, eating, speaking and walking will become worse over time. Depression is very common with a person that has Huntington's disease, and some people that have Huntington's disease are at a very high risk for suicide. Death usually occurs, when problems set in, like a fall or an infection that sets itself in the lungs." [8]

Lifestyle and Home Treatment

Huntington's disease will bring on a number of challenges that will require daily help. The following steps will help improve how a person with Huntington's disease feels:

A. *"They need to exercise regularly.* "This helps their physical and emotional health. Wearing well-fitting shoes will help improve their stability.

B. *Need to keep up with a good nutritional diet.* "A person with Huntington's disease may burn up as many as 5,000 calories in one day, so see that you get the right amount of nutrition to maintain your body weight, and see that you take extra vitamins and supplements. Because Huntington's disease can impair coordination, they may need help with eating, cutting food into small pieces or they need to pureed their food which makes swallowing much easier and will prevent them from choking. If you have Occupational Therapists come in they may make other suggestions on how to improve your loved ones swallowing. Use dishes and tableware that is made for people that have disabilities, this will help with the spills.

C. *Drink plenty of fluids*. People with Huntington's disease can become dehydrated very easy, and in the hot months they need to drink more liquids."[9]

Coping and Support

From the time that your loved one finds out that they have Huntington's disease, they need to work on the following.

A. "*Legal matters*. "Because Huntington's will affect their cognitive abilities," [10] they need to see that their wills and living wills are made up early in the course of the disease so their family will know how they wish to be taken care of at the end of their life.

B. *Arranging daily living assistance*. Most people with Huntington's disease sooner or later need help in performing daily tasks. They may want to live on their own but can't take care of the necessary tasks for independent living. In these cases, an assisted-living facility can provide a safe and comfortable living setting that allows them to maintain their independence.

C. *Emotional help*. Depression is common with Huntington's disease. Seek treatment from your doctor as soon as possible. "Ask your doctor if he or she knows of a Huntington's disease support group in your area. This may help you feel less alone, and they may be able to give you some tips on how to live with this disease. You can also call the Huntington's Disease Society of America, and they can let you know if there is a support group in your area; they also can give you information on the disease. They can be reached at 1-800-345-4372.

D. *Tips for caregivers.* Hire someone to come in and help care for the person with Huntington's disease. These people can do duties like light house work and fix meals; physical care of the person with Huntington's disease is one way to get help. You can also look and see what your state and federal health agencies have to offer in assisting for you and your loved one with Huntington's disease.

As the disease progresses, the person with Huntington's disease will no longer be able to live on their own. Long-term care facilities can help provide a safe and comfortable living situation for your loved one." [11]

Prevention

If there is a history of Huntington's disease in your family, you may want to look into genetic counseling before starting a family. If you do have the abnormal gene, you might think of adoption or other forms of reproduction assistance.

PARKINSON'S DISEASE

Definition

"Parkinson's disease is a progressive disorder of the nervous system that affects movement of the body. Parkinson's comes on little by little over time, often the disease starts with a hardly noticeable shaking in one hand. While shaking may be the most common symptoms of the disease, Parkinson's disease also brings on symptoms that can cause slowing or freezing of the body movement." [12]

"Family and friends may notice that your face is showing little or no expression and your arms don't swing when you walk." [13] They also notice that you are having a hard time with your speech, you are starting to mumble your words, and your voice is very soft and hard to hear. Parkinson's disease symptoms will worsen as the disease advances. There is no cure for Parkinson's disease, but there are medicines that can slow the symptoms of the disease down.

Symptoms

The symptoms can vary from person to person. They can start on one side of the body, and over time they will become worse, as symptoms begin to affect the other side of the body. Early symptoms can go unnoticed for a long time. Parkinson's disease has some of these symptoms.

A. *"Shaking or tremor*. A slight movement, in your body or your voice that cannot be controlled.

B. *Slowed movement.* Over time, Parkinson's disease will reduce your ability to move.

C. *Unbendable muscles.* The muscles will start to stiffen.

D. *Impaired posture and balance.* Our loved ones may become stooped as a result of Parkinson's disease. Balance problems also may occur, although this is usually in the later stages of the disease.
   1. Fall down
   2. Trip over things
   3. Have accident
   4. Collapse

E. *Loss of automatic movements.* A general characteristic of the motor system, that people can perform in their daily lives. A person that has Parkinson's disease will lose the ability to use their motor system in their lifetime.
   1. Blinking
   2. Smiling
   3. Swinging the arms when walking
   4. Fixed stare on their face
   5. Have a hard time with their speech

F. *Speech changes.* A person with Parkinson's disease may have speech problems as a result of the disease. They may speak softly, quickly, slur or hesitate before talking. They may also speech with a more monotone, them with the usual inflections.
   1. Start to speak softly
   2. Rapidly

3. Monotone
4. Slurring or repeating their words
5. Hesitating"[14]

Causes

"Researchers cannot find the exact cause for Parkinson's disease. They have found that the following does play a role in the disease:

A. Genes.
B. Environmental causes.
C. The lack of dopamine.
D. Low norepinephrine levels.
E. Presence of Lewy bodies." [15]

Risk Factors

The following are risk factors for Parkinson's disease:

A. "Age
   1. Parkinson's disease, generally begins when a person is in their 30's and older.
   2. The risk increase as a person gets older.
B. Heredity
   1. If you have a family member that has Parkinson's disease, you have a chance of developing the disease.
   2. The chances of developing Parkinson's is about 4 to 6 percent.
C. Sex
   1. Men are more likely to develop the disease
D. Exposure to toxins
   1. If a person is exposed to herbicides and pesticides, they have a higher chance of developing Parkinson's disease." [16]

Complications

A. "Depression
B. Sleep problems
C. Difficulty chewing and swallowing
D. Urinary problems
E. Constipation
F. Sexual dysfunction" [17]

Lifestyle and Home Remedies

"If the doctor has diagnosed you or your loved one with Parkinson's disease, you'll have to work with your doctor to find a plan for treatment that will help you find relief from your symptoms and have little side effect to the medicines, and changing your lifestyle will also help you live a better life with this disease." [18]

A. "Eat healthy
  1. Eat plenty of fruits, vegetables, and whole grains.
  2. Eating a balanced diet will provide omega-3.
  3. Take fiber supplement.
     a. Psyllium powder
     b. Metamucil or Citrucel
     c. Drink plenty of fluids daily
B. Walking to help balance
  1. Don't move too quickly.
  2. Put your heel to the floor first when walking.
  3. If you see that you are shuffling as you walk, stop and look at how you are standing.
  4. Try to stand straight.
C. Try to avoid falling:

    1. Don't pivot your body over your feet while turning. Instead, make a U-turn.

    2. Avoid walking backward.

D. Dressing

    1. Give yourself plenty of time to get dressed, so you will not feel as if you have to hurry.

    2. Always lay out your clothes, so you don't have to move too much around the room.

    3. Buy clothes that are easy to put on, like pants with elastic waistbands, dresses that are simple.

    4. Try to buy tops with fabric fasteners, like Velcro or snaps, which make dressing much easier for you or your loved one." [19]

Coping and Support

A. "Living with a disease can be very difficult; it is normal to be angry, depressed or discouraged over time. The disease can also be very frustrating when you try to walk, talk and even eating as the disease progress over time." [20]

B. Your family and friends are your best supporters with this disease. They should understand what is going on with you and the disease.

Prevention

"Since Researcher can't find what cause Parkinson's disease, finding ways to prevent the disease from coming into someone life is also difficult. But research has found that caffeine may reduce the chances of developing Parkinson's disease." [21]

WILSON'S DISEASE

Definition

"Wilson's disease is an inherited disorder that causes too much copper to collect in your liver, brain and other vital organs. Copper will play the key role in the development of healthy nerves, bones, and collagen and skin pigment. Copper is normally absorbed from our food, and any surplus is excreted through the bile, which is a liquid that is made in the liver.

"But people that have Wilson's disease, the copper isn't eliminated properly. Instead the copper accumulates in the liver, brain and other organs in the body. This can be life threatening to you or your loved one that has Wilson's disease. If the copper is left untreated, the disease can be very fatal, but if the disease is diagnosed early, a person can live a normal life."[22]

Symptoms

"Wilson's disease causes a wide variety of symptoms that can be mistaken for other diseases and conditions. Symptoms can be different, this depends on what parts of the body are affected by this disease.

The following symptoms are found in Wilson's disease

A. Clumsiness
B. Depression
C. Difficulty with speech
D. Difficulty swallowing
E. Difficulty walking
F. Drooling

G. Easy bruising

H. Fatigue

I. Involuntary shaking

J. Joint pain

K. Loss of appetite

L. Nausea

M. Skin rash

N. Swelling of arms and legs

O. Yellowing of the skin and eyes" [23]

Causes

"Wilson's disease occurs when a gene changes and leads to an increase of copper in the body.

A. How does the gene change occur?

    1. It is passed down from one generation to the next.

    2. "Wilson's disease is inherited as a chromosome producing feature. What this means is that you have to inherit two copies of the abnormal gene, one from each parent. To receive the disease, but if you only receive one copy of the gene, you are considered a carrier and can pass the gene down to your children.

B. How the gene changes cause Wilson's disease?

    1. "The changes that cause the disease occurs in a gene called ATP7B. When the changes occur in this gene, it leads to problems with a protein that's responsible for moving excess copper out of the liver. Where a person with Wilson's disease their gene will not remove

the excess copper from their liver, what it will do is to collect in other organs, like the brain, eyes and kidneys." [24]

Complications

A. "Scarring of the liver
B. Liver failure
C. Liver cancer
D. Lasting neurological problems
E. Kidney problems" [25]

Lifestyle and Home Remedies

A. "Doctor sometime recommends limiting the amount of copper in the diet during the first years of treatment. As the symptoms recede and the copper levels drop in the body, the person may be able to add some copper back into their diet.
B. This is a list of copper containing foods that is given to us by the Mayo Clinic.
    1. Look to see if vitamins and mineral supplements have copper in them.
    2. Liver
    3. Shellfish
    4. Mushrooms
    5. Nuts
    6. Chocolate
    7. Dried fruit
    8. Dried peas, beans, and lentils
    9. Avocados
    10. Bran products

C. Copper in tap water
  1. You need to have your pipes checked to see if you have copper pipes in your home. If you have a well, you need to have the water tested to see if the water has copper.
  2. If copper is in your pipes or well, don't drink the water, but use filtered or distilled water.
D. Copper pots and pans
  1. You should not use copper pots and pans to cook in.
  2. Do not store food in copper containers."[26]

VASCULAR DEMENTIA

Definition

"Vascular dementia is a term that describes impairment to our thought processes, which causes problems in the blood vessels that feed oxygen to the brain. In some cases, the blood vessels in the body may be completely blocked, which can cause strokes, but not all strokes are cause by vascular dementia. It will depend on how bad the stroke is and where the stroke occurred in the brain. Vascular dementia also occurs when the blood vessels in the brain become narrow or reducing the amount of blood flow to the brain. Vascular dementia has a range from 1 to 4 % of people that are over the age of 65. This is because there is no treatment for this disease." [27]

Symptoms

"The symptoms can vary; this depends on what part of the brain has been affected by the disease. Our loved ones that have been affected by this disease can experience these symptoms:

A. "Confusion and anxiety
B. Unsteady walking
C. Urinary frequency
D. Night wandering
E. Depression
F. Not able to organize thoughts or events
G. Having trouble planning ahead
H. Trouble communicating
I. Memory loss
J. Poor concentration"[28]

"Vascular dementia symptoms often come on little by little and will become worse over time, this can happen by a series of strokes or mini strokes. There are some forms of vascular dementia that can have the same symptoms as Alzheimer's disease.

Alzheimer's disease and vascular dementia can occur together. In fact, scientists believe that it's more common for these two diseases to occur together."[29]

Causes

Vascular dementia is most often caused by the following:

A. "Complete blockage of the blood vessels in the brain
B. Narrowing of the blood vessels in the brain
C. Low blood pressure
D. The brain hemorrhage
E. Blood vessels being damage from such disorders as lupus or temporal arteritis."[30]

Risk Factors

The following risk factors will not help vascular dementia from not coming into someone's life. So we need to see that the following are kept under control:

A. Increasing with age. *A person in their eighties and nineties are much more likely to have vascular dementia than a person in their sixties and seventies.*
B. "History of stroke
C. High blood pressure
D. Diabetes
E. Smoking
F. High cholesterol" [31]

Prevention

When you keep your blood pressure, diabetes, and cholesterol under control and also stop smoking, you have a better chance to prevent this disease from coming into your life.

LEWY BODY DEMENTIA

Definition

"Lewy body is the second most common type of progressive dementia after Alzheimer's disease. The reason that Lewy bodies diminish mental abilities of a person is that it may also cause visual hallucinations, which may take the form of seeing shapes, colors, people or animals that aren't there or, more complexly having conversations with deceased loved ones.

Another indicator of Lewy body dementia may include daytime drowsiness or periods of staring into space. Like Parkinson's disease, Lewy body dementia can result in rigid muscles, slowed movement and tremors. Like Alzheimer's disease, Lewy body dementia has abnormal buildup, which develop in areas of the brain that will make thinking and movement more difficult for the person with the disease."[32]

Symptoms

Let's look at some of the symptoms that take place in Lewy body dementia.

A. "Visual hallucinations, is one of the first symptoms that will be seen in Lewy body
B. Movement disorders
C. Delusions
D. Cognitive problems
E. Sleep difficulties
F. Fluctuating attention"[33]

"A person that has Lewy body can develop symptoms of Alzheimer's and Parkinson's within one year of each other."[34]

Causes

The cause of Lewy body dementia isn't known, but the symptoms may be related to Alzheimer's or Parkinson's disease.

A. "Lewy body has some of the symptoms that is linked to Parkinson's disease.
B. "Lewy bodies are often found in the brain of people that have Parkinson's disease and other dementias. C. For our loved ones that have Lewy bodies, their brain has the plaque that is associated with Alzheimer's disease."[35]

"Scientists tell us that Lewy body may have the same type of symptoms that is found in Alzheimer's disease. On the other hand, Lewy body and Alzheimer's can coexist in the same person."[36]

Risk Factors

Like any disease, there are always risk factors that take place. Well, Lewy body is no different. The risk factors are as follows:

A. "A person being over the age of sixty
B. Being a male
C. Having some one in your family that has Lewy body dementia"[37]

Complications

The difficulties that come with Lewy body are as follows:

A. "Lewy body progresses with time.
B. The following reason can bring complications to Lewy body
  1. Severe dementia
  2. Death, a person lives on the average of about eight years after being diagnosed"[38]

FRONTOTEMPORAL DEMENTIA

Definition

"The term *frontotemporal* is another name for the frontal and temporal lobes of the brain. This area is usually referred to the part of the brain that gives us our personality, behavior, thinking, and language. The section of the frontotemporal will waste away or shrink over time. Symptoms can vary from person to person, depending on what part of the brain has been affected. In some people the frontotemporal is an ongoing change in their personality, where others lose the ability to use and understand language.

Frontotemporal is often misdiagnosed as a psychiatric problem or Alzheimer's disease. This disease tends to appear at a younger age than Alzheimer's disease does; it falls between the ages of forty to seventy." [39]

Symptoms

"Identifying clearly which diseases will fall into the category of frontotemporal dementia presents a challenge to scientists. Symptoms will vary from one person to the next. Scientists have recognized several groups of symptoms that tend to occur in frontotemporal dementia. More than one symptom may be apparent in the same person. Over time the symptom of frontotemporal will get worse, and our loved ones will need twenty-four-hour care.

We will see some of these symptoms start to appear in our loved ones:

A. Behavioral changes
   1. More and more inappropriate behavioral will take place
   2. Loss of understanding and other relationship skill
   3. Lack of judgment and inhibition
   4. Lack of interest in life and people
   5. Compulsive behavior
   6. A decline in personal hygiene

      7.   Changes in eating habits
      8.   Lack of awareness of thinking or behavioral changes
  B. Speech and language problems
      1.   Shake
      2.   Inflexibility
      3.   Muscle spasms
      4.   Poor coordination
      5.   Difficulty swallowing
      6.   Muscle weakness" [40]

Causes

"A number of different genes have been linked to what can cause frontotemporal dementia from coming into someone's life. But more than half of the people who develop this disease will have no family history of frontotemporal dementia.

The parts of the brain that has been affected will take on the form of Pick bodies, this can happen in some cases of frontotemporal dementia. At one time frontotemporal dementia was known as Pick disease, but now we see that the temporal are now being affected by the abnormal protein that fills the nerves cells of the brain." [41]

Risk Factors

If your family has a history of frontotemporal dementia, there is a very high chance that you could develop the disease. There is no other risk factor that is known with this disease

POSTERIOR CORTICAL ATROPHY (PCA)

Definition

"Posterior Cortical Atrophy (PCA) is also known as Benson's syndrome, is the visual variant of Alzheimer's disease. PCA will cause shrinking to the back part of the brain. This will cause a person to have difficulty with their vision. Most people with PCA think that they need to see the eye doctor and have new glasses. See as we get older our vision starts to become impaired. But in people with PCA their visual problems are not with their eyes, rather it is the shrinking of their brain and this makes it hard for the brain to make sense of what information is being sent.

In the vast majority of PCA cases, the principal cause is Alzheimer's disease and the brain tissue that an autopsy shows is an abnormal buildup of proteins and tau that form plaques and neurofibrillary tangles as is seen in Alzheimer's disease. Although PCA is almost always caused by Alzheimer's disease, it can also be due to other diseases including dementia with Lewy bodies and Creutzfeldt-Jacob disease. PCA is thought to affect less than 5% of people with Alzheimer's disease, although the studies are lacking and PCA has been under-recognized in the past." [42]

Symptoms

A. "Blurred vision
B. Difficulties reading (particularly following the line of the text when reading)

C. Finding that letters appear to move around or become superimposed over one another
D. Writing with non-visual aspects of language preserved
E. Problems with depth perception
F. Sensitivity to bright light or shiny surfaces
G. Double vision
H. Difficulty seeing clearly, feeling that their eyes are jerking around or not completely under one's control.
I. Difficulty seeing clearly in low light
J. Having trouble reaching out to pick up an object
K. Having problems recalling how to spell words
L. Difficulties with handwriting
M. Difficulties with remembering shapes, letters and numbers
N. Problems dealing with money and small change
O. Difficulties using hand tools, like kitchenware, cutlery, scissors, and glasses
P. Having problems getting dressed" [43]

As the disease progresses, we will see other symptoms come into play.

A. "Getting lost while driving or walking in familiar places.
B. They cannot remember the faces of their family and friends or look at an object and tell what it is.
C. Judging distances.
D. Judging the speed of moving traffic.
E. Perceiving movement among things that are stationary.

F.   Rarely visual hallucinations.

G.   Calculation skills and the ability to make coordinated movements are affected in some cases."[44]

Progression

"This disease will affect people around the midfifties or early sixties when they will start to see symptoms. PCA is also found in more women then men. As the disease develops, the symptoms of Alzheimer's disease will start to show more with PCA. There is no definitive test that will tell us if a person has PCA. Some people live approximately the same length of time as individuals with Alzheimer's (on the average of tent o twelve years) where other can live with PCA for a long time." [45]

The sooner that we get the right diagnosis, the easier it will make it for us and the doctors to manage the disease. This will also help family members to see that their loved one's financial and legal affairs are in order for the future.

From the time that Dad was diagnosed (in 2002) with Alzheimer's, I had to find out all that I could about this disease so I could give him the best care when he came to live with us. Dad and Mom moved to South Carolina in March 2005, and had a home of their own. In August 2007 they had to move into our home for two reasons. Mom had a heart attack, and my husband was taking on a new job in Madison Indiana, and I was going to be doing all of the twenty four hour care by myself. Even though I had done a lot of research on Alzheimer's, I still was not prepared to handle this on my own. A person with Alzheimer's can be a handful at times. With Roger in Madison Indiana, Mom didn't like the idea that she and Dad were going to have to stay with me in South Carolina until our home sold, for her this was a very hard time in her life. With her husband having Alzheimer's disease, her oldest son (Roger) gone to start a new job, and the death of her second son (Craig) just a few months earlier, made her feel like her world was falling apart around her. As for Dad he just went with the flow at first. But there were days that he would flare up and get very angry at Mom and me. When these days would happen I had to be able to say to myself, that this is what God wanted me to do. Ephesians 6:2–3 said, "God tell us to care for our parents just like they cared for us when we were little" (NIV).

I knew by caring for Dad and Mom this was what God wanted me to do for them. This was also the way that God wanted me to be a good and obedient wife. Over the last twenty-seven years, I have come to look at my in-laws as my own parents. They had raised the man that I loved very much and have given him to me as my husband. It was my duty as a wife and daughter-in-law to care for them for the rest of their lives. Even though some days would be hard to deal with, I needed to keep in mind that throughout all of this, God had asked me to do this job, and I had to be obedient to Him first.

So I am recommending that when you have to care for your parents or in-laws, please do it for the man or woman that you love with all your heart. Also realize that you are doing what God has asked you to do.

I would like to speak to all the daughters- and sons-in-law for a little bit. Even though you might not get along with your mother or father-in-law, you need to know that taking care of your in-laws for your husband or wife will mean so much to them.

Even though Dad and Mom would give me problems, or Mom got mad at me for something, and started to yell at me, and I would retaliate back by yell also. Dad would start to put his hand into a fist and start to raise his hand like he was going to hit me. All I had to do was to pick up the phone and tell him that I was going to call the Sheriff. He would put his hand down and go sit in his chair and not move for the rest of the day. Dad knew that I meant what I said, and he knew that I would carry out the matter at hand, you have to remember. I was alone with no one to protect me if Dad did hit me. So scent I was good friends with the Sheriff he offered to see that I was safe. I knew that I had to put my differences aside and take care of Dad and Mom for Roger while he was working in Indiana, the day would come when we would both be together and we could care for his parents together. By helping my husband, seeing to his dad's needs, as well as helping care for his mom who was sick herself, with chronic obstructive pulmonary disease (COPD) as well as heart disease. I was able to have a better understanding of what Alzheimer's disease is all about. Based on my personal experience in caring for my father-in-law, I am able to help families have a better understanding about this disease.

So please remember that God is calling you to put your differences aside and look at how you and your husband or wife can become a team in caring for your parents or your in-laws that have Alzheimer's.

Like all disease, we are now going to see how symptoms, life expectancy, treatment, statistics, and cost come to play a very big role in the disease of Alzheimer's.

SYMPTOMS

Alzheimer's has symptoms that are divided into two categories:

1. Cognitive
2. Psychiatric

It is very important that we understand these two categories, so the behavioral problems that are caused by the loss of our thought processes are not treated with antipsychotic or anti-anxiety medications.

Cognitive is the process of acquiring knowledge by the use of,

A. *Reasoning.* The process of thinking about something in an intelligent sensible way in order to make a decision or form an opinion.
B. *Intuition.* The ability to know or understand something through your feelings, instead of by considering facts or proof.
C. *Perception.* The ability to understand and make good judgments about something.

   A person with Alzheimer's disease will lose the ability to receive, store, retrieve, transform and transmit information from their brain.

We can use this little saying that was given to me by Dr. Patricia Parmelee, Ph.D., who is the director of Psychology for the University of Alabama: "Last in first out."

It means the last to come into our mind is the first to be lost with Alzheimer's disease.

There are three major psychiatric symptoms that show up in a person with Alzheimer's:

1. Personality changes

    Irritability, A person with Alzheimer's disease will become very irritable at time and as the disease advance. Caregivers and family will see thing like touchiness, petulance, cantankerousness, tetchiness, bad temper.

    I like to tell you a little short story about how Dad would become easily annoyed with me or his caregiver (We had to hire someone to look after Dad when I had to go out for the day when Benjamin and Mom were sick.) when we had to get him dressed for an appointment as well as the day.

    One day I was getting Dad ready to go to the doctors, and all at once he started to yell at me and said that I was hurting him. (See Dad didn't like to have anything pulled over his head or have his arms pulled back to get his hand into the sleeve of his shirt.) I told Dad that we have to put the shirt over his head and then put his arm in the sleeve, so he could wear the shirt. As I explained why we had to put his head into the shirt first, and then put his arm into the shirt, he would cram down and within no time the yelling stopped, and I was able to finish getting him dressed for his doctor appointment. (One of the changes that I made in Dads wardrobe was to see that none of his shirts where pullovers. Dress shirts worked better for Dad. I also saw that the shirts were just a little bigger, so when he went to put his arms into the sleeves he didn't have to pull back so much.)

Lack of interest. A person with Alzheimer's has a very hard time keeping active on a daily basis. (See a person with Alzheimer's disease has a very short-term memory, so they can't remember from one minute to the next. So that is why lack of interest will occur in our loved ones life as this disease advances.)

So to understand why lack of interest came into Dads life is to understand that his short-term memory was lacking in him having the ability to be involved and active in the world around him. Dad figured out really early in life that I was the one taking care of him; he knew that I would see to whatever he needed. I had to try to make him do something on his own, like brush his teeth, and try to eat his meal.

Withdrawal & Isolation —is where a person with Alzheimer's disease may remove or separate themselves from the world.

Even though Dad was a very outgoing person when he didn't have Alzheimer's, as a person with Alzheimer's, he did withdrawal and isolated himself from the world.

One day I was taking Dad and Mom to the Department of Motor Vehicle (DMV) to have their driver's licenses changed.

Before we left the house for the DMV, Dad told me that we were not going to tell anyone about his condition, but we could tell the staff at the DMV only. Dad did not know that before he and Mom moved to South Carolina, I went to the police, our church, and our community to let them know that Roger's Dad had been diagnosed with Alzheimer's.

About two day before I was going to take Dad and Mom to the DMV, I went to the DMV myself and told them that my father-in-law had been diagnosed with Alzheimer's disease and asked what I needed to do to have them not give him his driver's license. They told me that everyone has the right to have a driver's license, but he would need to take the test on his own with no help.

The next day when we got to the DMV, I helped Dad to the table where he was to take the test, and then I told him that he was going to have to take the test without help, and that he was not to ask Mom for any help, because she had to take her test also. Dad kept looking at me and I kept telling him that I couldn't help, that he had to do the test on his own or he needed to give up his license and get an identification card instead. Within a few minutes Dad was back and told me that he will get the identification card. I helped him fell out the forms, and the ladies then asked him for his keys, and told him that he was not to drive anymore. From that day

Dad never asked for his key or got behind the wheel of their car.

That day was a long and hard day for Dad. See he really didn't want to even go to the DMV. (Like I said before a person with Alzheimer's has a very short-term memory. So they withdrawal & isolate themselves from the world is a normal way of life for a person with Alzheimer disease.)

2. Depression,

    Identifying depression in our loved ones that have Alzheimer's/dementia can be very hard to see, because Alzheimer's/dementia and depression have the same symptoms.

    As for Dad he did have depression symptoms. Like the apathy he had no interest in anything and wasn't willing to make the effort to try to do something. Dad loved to play golf, but as the disease progressed he lost interest in the game of golf, he withdrew himself from the world, and had a very hard time concentrating when someone was talking to him. As well as having a hard time using his memory to carry on a conversation if you asked him a question and needed an answer he wouldn't say anything to you but just stare at you.

3. Hallucinations and delusions

    A person with Alzheimer's disease will hear, see, taste, touch and even smell things that are not real to them. Hallucinations and delusions will mostly start in the middle stage of the disease.

It will also make our loved one become very upset and emotional which can cause them to have problems.

Hallucinations was one of the things that I saw in Dad when he would get frighten about something or just being in a place that he didn't know where he was. Anxiety would start to appear along with getting nervous, and you could see fear set into his eyes. Not only did he have anxiety as time went on he would start to become paranoid about what was taking place.

Once Dad had to go to the hospital, because the assisted-living facilities though he was having a stroke, and at the same time they had lost our phone number. So Dad had to spend the night in the hospital alone. The next day when they found our phone number I headed right over to the hospital to see about Dad and when I walked into his room I found him strapped to the bed and hallucinating about people being on top of the closet, who wanted to kill him. The first thing I did was to unstrap Dad and claim him down and let him know that I was now here and I was going to take care of him and stay with him, until I took him home. Then I told Dad that I had to go get the nurse and have a talk with her to find out what was going on, and when would we see the doctor. The nurse that was taking care of Dad told me that the reason that Dad was tied down was that he became very hostile when they were trying to take blood so they could find out if he really did have a stroke.

Dad kept hallucinating the whole time we were in the hospital. All I could do was try to keep him clam and keep telling him that I was trying my best to get the doctor to come in and see us so I could take him home. That seemed to keep him clam for a little while.

When I was able to get him back to the assisted-living facility, and back to his routine, Dad did fine. He took the hand of one of the caregiver, and walk off if nothing had happing.

The next day I went to checkup on him to see how he was doing, and speak to the resident RN director, on the paperwork that the doctor sent back with me. As we were talking, Dad was taking a little walk and I said hi, He looked at me and told me to get out of here, we took it to mean that he remember that I had been at the hospital with him and all he could remember was the awful time he had and how very upset he was. I knew that Dad couldn't remember that I wasn't the doctor or nurse that took care of him. I was a little taken back with the situation, the resident RN director told me this happen often and just give him some time to forget the whole ordeal, and that is just what I did.

We need to remember that what our loved one say or does is not them, it is the disease talking. So keep loving them with all your heart, they are still Dad and Mom. That same day I had a meeting with the resident

RN director as well as the resident doctor. The doctor from the hospital sent back with me paperwork that would increase Dad medicine to a point that would put him into a zombie state. We all made the decision that we would not increase Dad medicine, and that was the best decision we ever made for Dad.

LIFE EXPECTANCY

The life expectancy of a person with Alzheimer's disease is two to twenty years. On average people can live for eight to ten years from the time that they have been diagnosed with Alzheimer's or other Dementia diseases. The stage of the disease will determine, as well as their general health how long they will live with the disease of Alzheimer's/dementia.

My Father-in-law lived with the disease of Alzheimer's for fifteen years after he had been diagnosed with Alzheimer's.

Our loved one's with Alzheimer's disease are likely to develop the following heart attack, stroke, or pneumonia.

They are more likely to die from pneumonia; "Alzheimer's disease is among the top ten leading cause of death here in the United States" [46]and is on the rise.

On March 17, 2012 Dad past away from double pneumonia. He had to be put in the hospital for a prostrate condition, and within three day he developed double pneumonia and within a day he was gone to be with our heavenly Father. Today we all miss Dad and Mom. But we know that they are in a better place and Dad has his mine back and Mom can breathe once more.

TREATMENT

Right now, there is no treatment that will cure the disease of Alzheimer's.

"Researchers are still working on ways that they can slow, reduce or reverse the mental and behavioral symptoms of this disease. They are also trying to find ways to prevent the disease from ever coming into someone's life." [47]

"The United States Food and Drug Administration (FDA) has approved several drugs for treating of the disease of Alzheimer's.

1. *Aricept, donepezil hydrochloride*, This drug has been approved for early stages of the disease.
2. *Exelon, rivastigmine*. This has been approved for mild to moderate Alzheimer's.
3. *Razadyne, hydrobromide*. This has been approved for mild to moderate Alzheimer's.
4. *Namenda, memantine HCI*. This has been approved for moderate to severe Alzheimer's." [48]

Dad was on two of these medications. (Razadyne, and Namenda) most of his life. These medications didn't cure Dad from Alzheimer's. All they did was to help slow down Dad symptoms of the disease. Doctors will prescribe these medications by themselves or with each other.

STATISTICS

Statistics play a big role in knowing more about Alzheimer's as a disease. "In the United State right now there are about 5.1 million people that are affected by the disease of Alzheimer's.

"This disease is on the rise with more and more of the population aging and as the baby boomers come into old age. The chances of developing Alzheimer's will double, every five years after a person reaches the age of sixty five and older. This statistic is given to us by the National Institute on Aging." [49]

"As our country ages, Alzheimer's is on the rise. The number of Americans that are sixty five and older will double between the years 2010 and 2050, to 88.5 million people, that is about twenty percent of the American population. For those Americans that are eight-five and older, the disease will rise three-fold, to 19 million. This statistic is from the United State Census Bureau.

It is also estimated that a half million Americans that are younger than sixty-five will have some form of dementia that includes Alzheimer's as well." [50]

"One in eight Americans over the age of sixty-five will have the disease of Alzheimer's/dementia, and over 15 million (80%) Americans that are between the ages of thirty-five and up are becoming unpaid caregivers to their family members. It is also estimated that caring for a person with Alzheimer's/dementia will cost $200 billion in 2012, by 2050 it will be 1.1 trillion dollars. Medicare and Medicaid only cover about 70% of the cost of caring for a person with Alzheimer's/dementia, 17% come out of the pockets of family members, and 13% will come from medical insurance companies and other sources.

In 2011 it was estimated 17.4 billion hours of unpaid care, contributed to the nation economic value of over $210 billion dollars. It's also estimated that 21.9 hours of care is given by a caregiver per week, or 1,139 hours per year. With the care valued at $12.12 per hour Alzheimer's/dementia will cost approximately $210.5 billion dollars in 2011." [51] These facts and figures were brought to us from the Alzheimer's Association.

COST

"It costs the United States as a whole for taking care of people with Alzheimer's approximately $100 billion a year. Alzheimer's costs United States businesses more than $60 billion a year. This is because of the following problems that take place with having a loved one with Alzheimer's:

1. *Lost productivity.* Businesses are losing productivity, because caregivers have to take time off to care for a loved one, and caregivers may get sick from being on overload all the time.
2. *Insurance cost.* Because more and more people are being diagnosed with Alzheimer's, it is costing more to take care of them.

The yearly cost of taking care of a person with Alzheimer's is about $20,000 to more than $80,000. This depends on which stage of the disease the person is in. The cost of having a loved one with Alzheimer's is one of the highest financial expenses that a family can have. For an example,

Nursing home and assisted-living facility. These cost a family about $3,500 to $8,000 per month. The cost will depend on where you live and what your area is charging for care.

Insurance premium. The amount that comes out of the family expenses every month, and we can also expect our loved ones insurance premium to be increased every year.

Personal needs. Toothpaste, shampoo, body wash, wipes, diapers, men's razors, makeup for women.

Bills. Medications, insurance premiums, and clothing.

Medications. These can cost the family that has a loved one with Alzheimer's about $300 to $ 800 a month, depending on which stage the disease is in. The cost of medications is always on the rise."[52]

CAREGIVERS GET SICK THEMSELVES

There is one thing that takes place when you are taking care of your loved one that have been diagnose with Alzheimer's/dementia. It is caring for you (caregiver). I like to give you an example of what happen to me as I was caring for Dad and Mom.

Being a full time, wife, mother, daughter-in-law and a full time, (twenty four-seven) caregiver, as well as a part-time student, scent my body into a physical and emotional overload.

I had been on a full time world wind with seeing to my families care and making sure that my school works was done on time. (I was getting my BA in History and not going to bed till 1:00 pm or 2:00 pm every night.) By the time the semester ended my body was so tied, that I became sick, with the flue which send me to bed for a week.

When this would happen I had to rely on others to help me out with Dads care. (See Mom was sick herself and caring for Dad was way too much on her and her legs, my husband, Roger, worked out of town, and my sister-in-law lived in Texas, and like I said before my brother-in-law, Craig, passed away in February of 2007.) Having a caregiver come in was a little help for me when I was sick. There was one problem with this picture, she had to leave after she put Dad down for a nap, (about 1:00pm or 2:00pm) and from that time on I was the caregiver. That can be a big problem. Because you can't get the rest that your doctor told you that you needed. I tried to lay down when both Dad and Mom took a little catnap right before I had to get dinner. (Sometime that was about 5 minutes.) But it seemed to work for me and I just went to bed right after I got them down for the night.

TIPS FOR CAREGIVERS

Now we are going to take some time a talk about what it means to be a caregiver to a family member that has Alzheimer's/dementia disease.

Educating yourself about this disease will help you to be a better caregiver and your loved ones life will be better till God calls them home. You can educate yourself by reading books, attending workshops, asking your loved ones doctor questions and looking information up on the internet.

Most of my nights were spent looking up information on the internet, and reading books. I only called Dads doctor when I really needed to get information that I couldn't find in books or the internet.

Learn how to care for your loved one with Alzheimer's. I also had to learn what type of care Dad needed as well as Mom.

One of the first things that I needed to do was to see that our home was safe for them when they move in. As time went on I became familiar with Dad and Moms behavioral patterns, and how to handle them. Daily activities were the easy part to caring for Dad and Mom. We always found ways to keep them busy. Like playing games, reading, just getting dressed tuned into a game.

Understand what your loved one can do and have patience with them. We need to have patience with our loved one when they are trying to do something. Like get dressed, eating, playing a game, or just try to have a conversations with you, if they can. For Dad this was very hard for him.

You need to take time for yourself. Having time to myself was one of the things that I had a hard time seeing to, when I was caring for Dad and Mom, when Roger (my husband) was living in Madison Indiana for his job. But I would try to have friends over for dinner, as well as finding other interests that I would like to do, for example, take a walk with my husband, work on one of my hobbies, like sewing, crafts, and I try to write in my journal every day.

A support system is one of the best things that caregivers can have.

One of the things that I had was a good support system to help me through this time being a full time caregiver for Dad, as well as Mom. I had people like my husband, pastor and his wife, good friends, and Dads doctor. But most of all I needed to have the Lord in my life. The Lord was always with me twenty-four hours a day, and he never left me.

As a caregiver, you need to go to the doctor with your loved one.

When Dad moved to South Carolina I had no problem finding him a good doctor. I was seeing a Neurologist that was fantastic with me and the care that he gave me for my Epilepsy. So I knew that he would be good in handing Dad and his Alzheimer's disease. As a caregiver, I knew that I needed to build a good relationship with Dads doctor, and scent he was my doctor I knew that there would be fewer problems, and at the same time my doctor had worked with Alzheimer's patients before.

Ask for his office, when I made the appointment for Dad and told them that Dad had Alzheimer's disease. They asked me to make sure to bring in my health POA so they could talk to me about Dads appointment as well as seeing to all of the paperwork.

You need to see that their financial, legal, and long-term care plans are made ahead of time. One of the first thing that I did when Dad and Mom moved to South Carolina was to see that all of their financial, legal, and long-term care plans were made ahead of time, and put into place.

These are the things that I made sure were put into place before Dad Alzheimer's became too advanced.

Cost. We (Roger and I) made sure that Dad and Mom had all the money that they need to see to their care, as well as for the nursing home or assisted-living facility, when time came for them to need more around the clock care.

Because caring for a person with Alzheimer's/ dementia disease is very expensive on the person as well as the family. So by seeing that their finances are put in order, this will help take the stress off of you.

Power of Attorney (POA). See that you have someone in the family has your loved one's POA so when they are no longer able to care for themselves, you or another family member will be able to take care of their affairs.

This was the very first thing that I did, was to see that Dad and Mom's Power of Attorney (POA) was put into place right away. With Dads memory going day after day we needed to see that his POA's were in place, so we could give him the best care. First we had to make sure that Roger (Dads son) had all of his Dad POA's for financial, legal and health. Second was to see that I had POA for just health, since I was going to be taking Dad to see the doctor, and I was going to be filling and signing all of his paperwork. As for Mom we made sure that all of her POA were put into place as well. We would not put her POA into action till she got very sick in 2010.

Long-term care. Look into what it will cost your family when the time comes for you to move your loved one into a nursing home or assisted living.

After I took care of Dad and Mom financial, legal affairs, the next step was to look into long-term care for Dad. (As we move more into the book we will come to a chapter on long-term care. Here we will talk about how to make it easier to transition into residential care, as well as how to plan and paid for residential care.)

Loss of income. Will someone in your family lose their income by having to stay at home and care for your loved one?

I wasn't able to go to work, and bring in more income for my family, because now I was needed to stay home and take care of Dad and Mom.

Housing costs. Will you have to move your loved one into your home? Will you have to buy a new home that is safer and does not have stairs? Will your new home be closer to the doctor's office? Will you have to make modifications to your home, like, new locks, rails, safety devices, wheelchair ramps? Or do you even have to renovate a room for your loved one?

As for us, when Dad and Mom moved in with us. We had to make sure that our home had hand rails from their apartment to the house, rails in the bathroom, night light all thought the house at night. (When I say night light I mean little lamps that hold a 25 watt bulb.) We also re-arranged our home to add Dad and Mom belongings to make them feel welcome, loved, and a part of our family. Even though this move would be hard on all of us, (my family and Dad and Mom) we would all make it through this time in our lives. Because of one thing "we are family."

Medical costs. Will you need someone to come in and care for your loved one, if you care for your loved one at home, use adult day care? Or will your loved one have the financial needs for their hospital bills and doctor bills? Does your loved one have the right medical insurance? Will you have to pay for their medications, personal needs, and other things they will need as this disease progresses?

Be in a good mood. Try to put some humor into your loved one's life. Talk to them about the past, like their family, school, church, jobs, and the places they have been to and seen in their lifetime. Give them a hug to let them know that they are safe and loved. And most of all enjoy your relationship with your loved one while you are still able.

There was no problem seeing that humor was put into our home. Mom loved the tell jokes and laugh. But for Dad he didn't like it when we would get loud and have a good time. He would, get mad, or walk away and close the door to his apartment. After sometime, that Dad had been in our home he knew that we weren't going to stop having fun. He had to join in or go to his room.

Even though you have a loved one with Alzheimer/ dementia living in your home, it doesn't mean that you have to stop living. God made us to have fun on His earth.

PUTTING TOGETHER A DAILY ROUTINE FOR A PERSON WITH ALZHEIMER'S

By putting together a daily routine for Dad, this also helped make his and my day much easier to handle, and it also kept him busy most of the day. I hope this daily routine will give you some ideals to uses with your loved one.

Getting up for the day.
Dad was up by 8:00 a.m. to start his day.
Bathroom break.

Breakfast.
Before I or the caregiver would wake up Dad, we would have his breakfast made and ready for him.

Bath.
While he was having his breakfast, one of us (Caregiver or I) would get his bath ready, see that his clothes were laid out for the day, put toothpaste on his toothbrush, have his shaving things out and ready for him to use. I would also make sure that the bathroom was nice and warm for Dad and that we had laid out

towels and washcloth for him. We also made sure that the body wash was where he or us could get to it easy.

I always gave Dad a bath in the morning, because Dad had a hard time with the sun beginning to set about 6:00p.m. Dad would start to get paranoid about the day coming to an end. There is something about the sun setting that has an effect on some people that have Alzheimer's disease.

A person with Alzheimer's does not like change in their life. They like to do the same things over and over. Remember that if you say that you are going to do something, please follow it through. Your loved one with Alzheimer's does not understand why you are changing your mind, and they become very confused on what is going on.

Getting dressed for the day.

After Dad had his bath, it now was time to get dressed, brush his teeth, and shave.

Have a little time to rest from bath and getting dressed.

This was hard work for Dad.

Do morning activities.

Have a walk, look at family pictures to see if I could bring back a memory and talk with Dad about his life as a child. (This can be whatever you like to do. We always did something simple in the morning, because Dad bath made him very tied.)

Bathroom break.

Morning snack about 10:00 a.m.

Lunch about 12:00 p.m.

About 11:30 a.m. we would fix Dad's lunch and set the table so it would be ready for him at 12:00 p.m.

Bathroom break.

Nap about 2:00 p.m.

While he was taking his nap, I would do some housework or school work and have some time to myself. This was also the time that the caregiver would head home for the day, and I took over for the evening.

Up from his nap.

I would see that he was up by 3:00 or 3:30 p.m. so he could go to bed on time.

Bathroom break.

Afternoon snack about 4:00 p.m.

Afternoon activities.

We would go for a walk, or I would get Mom to talk to Dad. So I could get dinner. (This can be whatever you like to do.)

Bathroom break.

Dinner about 6:00 pm.

After dinner,

Dad took a walk with Mom around the yard.

Evening activities.

Watched a little television or Dad and I would read a little from his Bible before bed.

Evening snack at about 8:00 pm.

Bathroom break.

Bedtime about 9:00 p.m.

Dad did not sleep well when he lived with us because Mom always kept the television on twenty-four hours a day. She would not come up into our living room when

Dad was taking his nap or go to bed for the night. She told us that she needed the television on for her to fall asleep. Yet this made it hard for Dad to get a good nap or a good-night's sleep.

It is recommend that the television is put in another room, and this will let the person with Alzheimer's sleep better. Also this will reduce behavioral problems.

CAREGIVERS NEED TO HAVE SOME PERSONAL TIME

Having a vacation is very important to a caregiver. This is a time where a caregiver can have some time to themselves and be able to put themselves back on track and not just focus on their loved one's care.

In this part of our family story, I wish that I had had family members to give me a break more often. Camille lived in Texas and had financial problems that made it impossible for her to come and give me some time off. Craig could not help since he passed away. So I knew that I was going to have to find other ways to have some time off from caring for Dad.

One of the ways that I could get some time off was to see if Benjamin (my son) would be able to look after his grandparents at night and made arrangements with a caregiver service for the day time. The caregiver service would come in till Benjamin got home from school, and when he had to go off to work at 4:30 p.m. (Benjamin had an after school job when he was in high school.)

The only thing with caregiver's services is they cost $100 or more a day. But they are worth every penny.

Having a caregiver was a blessing to Dad and me. She gave me time for myself, and when she left for the day, I was ready to take over and care for Dad. I had the caregiver services stay on after I came back from my time off. I like the lady that was coming to take care of Dad and I could use the help with Roger working out of state. Mom wouldn't have to step in and care for Dad, when I was out for the day or on vacation.

To make life easier for Mom, I would see that meals were made and placed in the freezer, and all she or Benjamin had to do was to take the meal out in the morning, and warm them up at dinnertime, and this would give everyone a good and healthy meal.

At the same time when Benjamin had to go off to work, our neighbors were so kind to keep an eye on Dad and Mom until he got home from work. (That was about 11 p.m.) My neighbors knew that I needed to see to my health. I need to share with you something, that our neighborhood never gave a second thought. "God tells us to love our neighbors as ourselves." That verse was part of our neighborhood and we lived it every day.

The vacation also gave me some time to be with my friends, to communicate with other people, see what the world has to offer me, and let me grow in other ways than just as a caregiver for Dad and Mom. I need to remember that I was a person and I have the right to do something for me. Putting one day a week aside for myself, and let others come in and care for Dad and Mom. This also lets them see how much work it takes to care for a person with Alzheimer's, and how this disease has affected our family.

HOW TO LOOK FOR A GOOD IN-HOME CAREGIVER'S SERVICES

Like all families that have a loved one that has been diagnosed with Alzheimer's, we didn't want to place Dad into an assisted-living facility right away; we want to keep him home with us as long as we were able to. As the disease begins to advance in Dad, we knew the day was coming that we would need more care for Dad.

A caregiver or services would be able to help us with Dad needs. The caregiver or services that I was looking at need to be interviewed to see if they were the right fit for caring for Dad. These are some of the questions that I used in my interview with the caregivers or the services that I was looking at for Dad care.

I ask them the questions over the phone to the caregiver's services before I used their agency in Dad care. As for the caregivers that the agency would send me, I copied the questions and ask them to please fill out and answer all the questions that applied to them. Then we went over, so I could make sure that they were telling the truth.

I need to make sure that I was getting Dad the best care, and I also need to make sure that abuses would not occur to Dad when I would be away from the house for the day. With Mom when she had an appointment with her doctors.

1. Your name, address, home and cell phone numbers?
2. What time of the day is the best time to call?
3. Do you smoke?

4. Do you have a driver's license? If yes, do you have transportation and car insurance?

5. How far do you live from our home?

6. Have you been trained in CPR or first aid?

7. Have you been trained in the behaviors of dementia care?

8. Do you keep your training up to date, like once a year?

9. Can I have your permission to run a background check?

10. Do you understand the duties that this position will require of you?

11. Are you able to work full-time and overtime when needed?

12. Do you have any health problems that will prevent you from lifting heavy object?

13. Will you be able to transfer our loved one from a wheelchair to their bed or a car?

14. Will you be able to fix meals for our loved one?

15. What type of cooking do you do? (Some loved one only like Southern or Northern cooling.)

16. Have you ever cooked for older people?

17. How do you feel about caring for an elderly or disabled person?

18. How do you feel about caring for a person with Alzheimer's or dementia disease?

19. How would you handle a person who has hallucinations and delusions?

20. How would you handle a person that become emotional, has mood swings often, is nervous all the time, can become frightened much easier,

is restless more often, and can be angry much easier? What type of training do you have in these areas?

21. What type of people have you cared for?
22. Can you give me an example of a difficult situation that you had to handle on your last job?
23. What time commitment are you willing to make to stay on the job?
24. Where was your last job?
25. How long were you there?
26. Why did you leave?
27. May we contact your past employer?
28. May we have your employer's name, phone number, and e-mail address?
29. Are you willing to keep daily records?
30. Do you know how to use a computer?
31. When will you be able to start working for us?
32. Why should we hire you for this job?
33. Are you willing to sign a contract saying that you will not accept anything from our loved ones?
34. How will you keep the family informed daily?
35. Can you give us two job references and one personal reference?

TIPS FOR THE HOLIDAYS

Holidays can be one of the hardest times for a person with Alzheimer's. They can't handle lots of people in the same place at the same time. They do not understand what a holiday is and why we celebrate that holiday.

Communicate concerns. This is a good time to have a good talk with your family about sharing the responsibilities of caring for your loved one that has Alzheimer's. By sharing the responsibilities with each other, you all will have a better life, no one will have caregiver burnout, and sharing the responsibilities will also bring your family closer together in having a better understanding of what this disease will do to your loved one.

This is a good time for me to jump in and tell you how I handled telling our family and friends about Dad having Alzheimer's and how we all need to share the responsibility for his care. When Dad and Mom were getting ready to move to South Carolina, I told my husband (Roger) that he would have to have a talk with his brother about coming every other month to help us with Dad's care. But they only wanted to come once a year. I had to explain to my brother- and sister-in-law that Alzheimer's is a family disease, and we all have to do our part, and one person can't do this job all by themselves. As for Roger's sister since she lives in Texas, financial problems and was a single mother coming once a year would make it more difficult on her to come to help out with her parents. So we would send Mom to see her daughter and grandsons and give them some time to see and enjoy themselves, and at the same time this give me a little time off to recharge my battery.

When you are the only caregiver in your family who is caring for a person with Alzheimer's and your husband is living out of town because of his job, you will need all the help that you can receive from your friends and family.

So if you are the only person in your family that is caring for a person that has Alzheimer's, *please* know that God is pleased with what you are doing for your loved one.

Set realistic expectations. You need to take a good look at what your loved one is capable of handling with large groups of people around the holiday times.

Dad went into overload when we all went to see Craig's family when he got sick with cancer. I was not thinking about how this was going to affect him. We were not in the house for more than a minute when Dad started to get nervous, he could not stand the noise of everyone talking all at once. (Loud noises make a person with Alzheimer's become uneasy and nervous with the world around them.)

At the same time I had a paper that I needed to be working on and was not able to keep an eye on Dad like I normally do, I thought that everyone would watch Dad for me, and I also thought that they knew how very important my paper was for school.

You can tell that people do not look at caring for a person with Alzheimer's the same way that you do. Everyone was having a good time, and no one was watching out for Dad. After an hour, I went to see how Dad was doing; I found him heading out the back door. I asked Dad where he was going; he said that he was going home. "This place is too noisy."

I asked Roger to take both of us back to the hotel so I could put Dad down for a nap and work on my paper for school. This would also get Dad out of the noisy house, and everyone could continue having a good time and not have to look after Dad.

When we got back to the hotel, I told Roger that the next time the family wanted to get-together, they were going to have to do it without Dad and me. He would have to take time off from work to bring his mother to see his brother when she wanted to see him.

Roger said it was not fair for me to have to stay home all the time with Dad. I told him that when we signed on for this job, someone was going to have to stay with Dad and since Craig was sick and not able to come to our home and Mom wanted to see her dying son more that I was going to have to be the one to stay home with Dad. Roger told me that he loved me very much and thanked me for caring so much about his Dad. Someone has to care for the person that has Alzheimer's, they can't care for themselves.

Select appropriate activities for the holiday. When it comes to putting holiday activities together for your loved one try to have them take part in singing holiday songs, decorating the Christmas tree, or even help wrap Christmas gifts. This is also a good time to bring out family memories like pictures, and heirlooms.

When you are talking to your loved one about your family memories do not ask them who is in the picture or do they know who the heirlooms belonged to. Rather you say to them Dad I did not know that your mother was so beautiful. You do the memory stimulation.

The same goes for when you are opening gifts from each other. Give your loved one just one gift at a time. Let me explain: my husband's family loved to give everyone their gifts all at once, and open all of their gifts at the same time. You can have everyone open one gift at a time, have someone help your loved one with their gifts, and read the gift tag to them, by doing this your loved one will enjoy Christmas a lot more.

I found when Mom, Roger, or I helped Dad with his gifts and told him who had sent or was giving the gift to him, he then enjoyed opening Christmas gifts more. By doing things little by little with Dad, it made the holiday a lot more enjoyable for him and me. Also if your loved one gets tired from opening gifts, you can stop and go on to another activity.

When your family understands why the holidays bring anxiety and behavior problems to your loved one, the whole family will come to have a wonderful Christmas that you all can remember for the rest of yours and your loved one's life.

Pare down traditions. With the holiday and religious observances and taking care of a loved one with Alzheimer's, you might become overworked. If you find that you cut back on some of the observances, you will feel a lot better and be able to enjoy the holiday more.

One of the things that we did was to see if Mom would stay with Dad while we were out for an evening. Roger and I also made it a point to only go to about two events. I also made it a point to have Dad eat his dinner and get ready for bed before I left for the evening. This made things a lot easier on Mom while we were out. I would also ask someone to look in on them, and I would call her throughout the even to see how thing were going.

Adapt family gatherings. One thing that makes a person with Alzheimer's have more behavioral problems is having too many people over at the same time. People with Alzheimer's do not like to have their day interrupted, and their mind can't handle change.

Instead of having the whole family at the same time and on the same day, see if you can have each family come on different days. This will make it much easier for your loved one to handle family gatherings, noise, and their routines will not be altered.

For instance, the time we went to see Craig when he got sick back in October 2006, I could have asked Camille and her boys to come to our home so she could see her Dad, after she had gone to see her brother. This would have made life much easier on Dad.

Stick with familiar settings. Taking your loved one out of their environment can cause them to become very confused about where they are. For example, if your loved one has a hard time going to church on Sunday, see if you can take them to an earlier service, or if you can ask your pastor to come to your home and have prayer with your loved one.

When Mom was put into the hospital, Dad had a hard time dealing with her being gone. Dad would not go to church or even go to the hospital. I asked our pastor if he would make a house call. He told me that was no problem. On Sunday afternoon he came over to pray with Dad.

So please remember to look at how your loved one is feeling and can they handle what is going on in their environment that day.

Head off problems. A person with Alzheimer's should not partake in alcohol at any time. Alcohol can cause depression; the risk of falling, and can add to brain cells loss.

Dad didn't drink alcohol.

Sundown can have a big affect on your loved one that has Alzheimer's.

Dad did have a very hard time when it came to the sun setting at the end of the day. So what I used to do was to see that all the drapes were closed about 4:30pm, so Dad wouldn't see the sun setting for the day.

That is why family visits for the holidays should be done earlier in the day. The sundown affect takes place in the middle stages of the disease.

As for family coming for a visit that was no problem. Most of the time it was just my family that Dad saw every day. Camille lived in Texas, Craig had passed away, and Craig children, lived to far away which make it very hard for everyone to try to make it for the holiday.

One of the other things that I did not do around the holidays was not to re-arrange the house. I knew that I had to be very careful, that I put the Christmas decoration in a safe place where Dad would not fall. I also had to look at Dad as a blind person or a little child that is just starting to walk, you would not want to put things where they can fall and hurt themselves.

When decorating your home for the holidays, be careful not to put decorations out in the walkway, see that the tree is placed in a corner of the room, do not hang decorations from ceiling lights or fans. Candles can make your loved one become scared; they do not understand open flames. So it is best to keep candles unlit for the holidays, or you can use candles that run on batteries that are safer.

When I started to put the Christmas decoration out, the first thing I did was to look at the house and see where to place the tree, what type of lights we are going to use, how many other decorations were we going to put out around the house. I knew that I had to make it as easy as possible for Dad to get around the house and not fall. I saw to it that the lights were mix colored so Dad could enjoy the holidays. (See white lights can make a person with Alzheimer's disease get very upset, and white lights are also very bright, where colored lights would calm Dad down so he would be able to enjoy the holidays.)

Rethink gift giving. One of the things that I did for Dad was to think of what type of gifts he had given Mom over the years, and what type of gifts they could pass down to their children, grandchildren, and great-grandchildren.

The first year that Dad and Mom were living with us, I had a charm bracelet made up from Dad. When the bracelet was finished, Dad went with me to the store to pick up the bracelet, and he could see his gift he was giving his bride. At the store, he told me that I did a good job. Knowing that this gift would mean a lot to Mom this Christmas, this was also the first Christmas that Dad was not able to buy a gift for her on his own. I was glad to help him out, knowing how much this would mean to the both of them.

Welcome youngsters. When it comes to children in your family, keep in mind that your loved one can have problems with little ones playing with their Christmas gifts, and they can also become very noisy and excited about the holidays.

What you need to do before the family gets together for the holidays is to call them and have a talk about how Dad or Mom will feel about having children around. Instead of having the whole family at the same time and on the same day, see if you can have each family come on a different day throughout the holiday seasons, and those that have young children ask them to only stay for about hour and a half. If the children are well behaved, they can stay a little longer. If the children are too noisy and will not quiet down, it would be better to take the children home early. You need to understand that noise can make Dad or Mom very uneasy.

Please keep in mind that you have to understand that your loved one with Alzheimer's does not understand what little children are like. I know that having a loved one with Alzheimer's makes for a lot of changes in your family. You must understand that this disease is turning Dad or Mom back into a child themselves.

Because our family lived in Texas, North Carolina, and California, having little one around wasn't a problem in our family. So the holiday's where very peaceful for Dad, all we had to do was to see that the day went very slow and he did fine with the holidays.

Joining a support group is one of the best things that you can do for yourself.

These are people that have gone through the same thing that you are going through. It is here that you can vent out your problems that you are having with your family, and your loved one that has Alzheimer's.

My support group was my family, church, and friends. They were always there for me.

Enjoy yourself. One of the things that you need to do around the holidays is to see if you can have a family member, friends, or caregiver services to come in and keep your loved one company so you can have some time to do your Christmas shopping, see old friend, go out to lunch or dinner with a friend or just have some time for yourself so you can enjoy the holidays just as well as everyone else. You love your loved one very much but they can be a handful, and they do not always understand that you need time to just be you and have fun.

This was one of the things that I didn't have when I was taking care of Dad and Mom. See my family didn't live close by, and weren't able to help me out with Dad and Mom. I understood what it felt like, not to be close to my parents. They lived with my sister in New Jersey, and I could only go to see them when I had the money, to pay the air fare. So please have some understanding with your family when they can't come and help or give you a little time to yourself.

COMMUNICATION

When communicating with a person or your loved one that has Alzheimer's disease, you need to remember that this disease will diminish your loved ones ability to communicate with the world. The following tips will help you to understand why we need to become good listeners to our loved ones.

1. *Remember that your loved one has emotions:* Keep in mind that your loved one might be feeling confused, anxious, sensitive, depressed, or suffering from low self-esteem.

   As Dad's caregiver communication was one of the hardest things to do with Dad. As his Alzheimer's advance more over the years the family and I had to be very careful with Dad's emotions when we were speaking to him.

2. *Using the five Ss',*

   As Dad's caregiver, I used the five Ss' method of speaking (Simple, Slow, Show, Smile, and Speak) to communicate better with him. By using the five Ss Dad was able to have a better time with his family as we all communicated with him on a daily bastes. So by trying to use these five Ss, you will be able to see how much fun it will bring your loved one in the world of communication.

A. *Simple*. Use simple words and sentences when talking or giving your loved one instructions. Please give your loved one instructions one step at a time.

B. *Slow*. Speak slowly and give plenty of time for your loved one to understand what you have to say or ask of them.

C. *Show*. Use body language to show what you want them to see. For example, use facial expressions, body movements, point to objects that you want your loved ones to see.

D. *Smile*. Smiling shows your loved one that you are friendly, kind, and loving.

E. *Speaking*. Your tone of voice needs to be calm, supportive, encouraging, and comforting when you are talking to your loved one.

By using the five Ss, our visits were fun and full of love for Dad. Even though he didn't communicate with us, we could see him light up and enjoy our visits.

When approaching your loved ones do it from the front where they can see and hear you. You do not want to speak to them from their back; this will frighten or upset them.

3. *Approaching* Dad from the front was a must when I would go to see him, and asking him if I could touch him to give him a hug or kiss. If I just went up to Dad and gave him a hug, he would get mad and push me way, and our visit was not a long visit. But if you did what he liked and approached him in the right way and

asked him "can I give you a hug or kiss". Then he would enjoy my visit and didn't want me to leave.

4. *When addressing:* You should always address your loved one by their name first. This will get their attention. and at the same time keep eye contact with your loved one.

By addressing Dad by his first name would always get his attention and he was able to understand what I was saying to him. I always addressed him as Dad, were other people that were not family addressed him as Mr. Richard or Mr. Johnson, and Dad was able to tell the difference between the two ways that he was being addressed.

5. *How to ask a question.* Only ask one question at a time, let there be some time between the question and the answer. and if your loved one does not seem to understand your question, repeat the question by using the same words.

When asking Dad question I would let there be time between the question and answer. But with Dad that never happen. See Dad wouldn't talk to anyone, all he would do was nod or just move his head.

6. *How to have a discussion.* Have your discussions in peace and quiet so your loved one will be able to hear what you are saying to them.

Avoid statements that sound negative.

We tried not to use negative statement with Dad, because negative statements would bring out negative emotions. I like to give you an example, when Dad's baby sister passed away. Sometime that week after Aunt Barbara passed away, Mom went to visit Dad.

She wasn't in his room for more than a minute than she told him that his sister had died.

I had told her earlier that she wasn't to say anything to Dad about Aunt Barbara passing away. Well that's not what she did, she went right on and told Dad. That afternoon, the assisted living facility called me at work, and told me that Dad was crying uncontrollably. At the same time they told me that my mother-in-law and husband had come to see him before lunch. I knew right away what had happen. I got off work early and went to have a talk with Dad, to see if I could calm him down.

I knew that Dad only remembered Aunt Barbara as a five year old little girl. He couldn't remember that she was a mother, grandmother, and a great grandmother as well, and that the Good Lord thought that it was time for her to come home where He could heal her. Once I explained this to Dad he started to feel better and stopped crying.

When I got home I had a talk with Mom and told her that she was never to tell Dad anything about someone passing away, at the same time my husband made the statement that we were never going to tell Dad when a member of our family passes away, he ask his Mom to please do this and have some understanding about Dad's emotional state, when it comes to family.

We never told Dad that Mom had passed away. But I know in my heart that he did know that Mom was gone to be with the Lord.

The next day I made sure that I went to see how Dad was doing, before I went to work. Dad had forgotten what happen the day before. This made me feel better and I knew that Dad was back to his old self.

7.   *Keep on talking, even if your loved one is no longer verbal.* When you keep talking this shows your loved one that you love and care for them.

That is the one thing that my family and I did when we went to see Dad. Even though he wasn't talking anymore, we all would keep telling him what was happening in the life of our family. See even those your loved one has Alzheimer's disease, they are still part of your family and they have the right to know what is going on in their family. We would tell Dad things like, when he had a new Great Grandsons, Emory, Everett, or his daughter was coming to see him and she was bring her new husband for him to meet, as well as Camille's son was also coming to see him to. Dad loved to have company, even though he didn't say much.

8.   *When you have to tell your loved one that they have Alzheimer's disease.* Please ask the doctor to be with you when you go to tell your loved one and their spouse about the disease of Alzheimer's.

Having the doctor with Camille made it easier to tell Dad and Mom that Dad had Alzheimer's disease. When Dad and Mom moved to South Carolina I took Dad to see a new doctor and we made sure that both Dad and Mom understood what was happing to Dad and the disease of Alzheimer's. Like always I had lots of questions for the doctor, he was willing to answer all of my questions. The doctor knew that I was going to be taking care for Dad and I also had to understand what the disease does to a person life.

You need to be honest with your family and friends, about your loved one having the disease of Alzheimer's. You also need to keep the doctor up to date on what is happening at home with Dad and Mom. When you have to tell your parents something that you know will make them upset, think first and be mindful of their feelings.

DAILY ACTIVES

As a caregiver there was one thing that I always made sure that Dad did in his day. That was to have some type of daily activity that would help stimulate his memories. As Dad moved into the assisted-living facility, (Ashton Gables) I knew that there would be more daily actives for him to take part in. But as always Dad was one not to do daily actives. It took tooth and nail to get Dad to do anything.

So let's take a look at how art actives can be good to do with your loved ones that has Alzheimer's/dementias.

My friends and the staff of Ashton Gables was kind enough to share with me some of the actives that they used with their residents on a daily basis.

ART

Art is a way to help bring out the imagination in our loved ones. There are many different types of things we can do through art.

1. *Keep it simple.* By keeping the art project simple your loved one will come to enjoy themselves, and not become frustrated with what they are doing and give up on the project. We can do things like painting,sculpting or making a picture book that can be use when you have to take your loved one to the hospital or a doctor's appointment.

2. *Evoke memories.* Bring back their childhood memories by drawing picture from the past.

3. *Play it safe,* as a caregiver check all labels and only buy paints and other materials that are nontoxic. You can also make your own paint and clay from ingredients that can be eaten. We have to remember that our loved ones will not be able to tell the difference between toxic and nontoxic materials. So it's up to us to see that all art materials are safe to use.

4. *Select stimulating materials.* When your loved one gets into the middle to late stage of the disease, they will respond best to bright colors of paints, homemade clay, and objects like candy boxes, balls of yarn. Looking at old photographs, and papier-mâché is also good for your loved one to use in an art activity.

5. *Create a comfortable setting:* Create a comfortable setting for your loved ones, and family members to enjoy as they work on their art actives, and help stimulate your loved ones memory. Let's look at some ways that we can create a comfortable art setting.

   Playing music in the background, this will relax everyone as they work on their art project remember to have good lighting, not too bright.

6. *Be positive.* Please use words like great job and terrific.ect.

7. *Talk about the artwork.* Talk about the artwork with your love ones, this will help you to spark a

conversation in your loved one. And at the same time please only ask open-ended questions.

8. *Start a gallery.* After your loved one has finished with their artwork, it will be nice to put it up where family and your loved one can see it. You can hang the artwork in places like the refrigerator and hallway, or if they are living in a long-term care facility, you can place their artwork in their room or the hallway outside their room; you can also make a photo book where you can keep all of your loved ones artwork.

Art can also be a good way that they can work on their motor skills, as well as physical rehabilitation, and art active can also bring them out of their shell. Art active can also bring the whole family together for family time, helps young children to have a good time and get to know their grandparents, and most of all shows young children that they do not have to be afraid of a person with Alzheimer's/dementia.

As for Dad, when it came to art activities, he had no interest in art. But one day the activity director at Ashton Gables was working with Dad, and out of the blue she got him to paint a picture. Today I have that painting hanging in my office. When I look at that painting I remember how difficult it was to get Dad to do any type of activity when he was at Ashton Gables. Most men have a very hard time doing art, music, or storytelling activies.

MUSIC

Music has the power to spark compelling outcomes even in the late stages of Alzheimer's.

When music is used appropriately, the activity will help our loved ones with their mood swings, manage stress, anxiety, worry, nervousness, and depression.

Music can also take them back to their childhood.

I would like to stop here and talk to you about music; we as caregivers need to remember that our loved one will not like loud music or when we raise our voice about something. Raising our voice or playing loud music will make them think we do not like them or they have done something wrong. Loud music will also hurt their ears, making them upset.

Let's take a look at four ways that music can work with our loved one.

1. *Music associations.* Most people that have Alzheimer's/dementia can relate to music. This is why music activities will play a very big part in the life of a person with Alzheimer's disease. We want to keep their memory open to their world. Most people with Alzheimer's can remember important events that have taken place in their lifetime though music.

   If a particular song was played Dad emotions would start to come out and tears would start to flow, because this song brought back his childhood, the time he and Mom were a young married couple. All we (Ashton Gables and I) could do was to let time take its course, and by the next day Dad was back to his old self.

2. *Sound of music.* Music can also help with their daily routine. Here are some songs that Ashton Gables used with their residents:

A. Stimulative music is more a quiet and quick tempos that will have your loved one clapping their hands and tapping their feet. Dad was always clapping his hands and tapping his feet all day long at the assisted-living facility. This is one of the ways that we knew that he was happy, and full of life. Assisted-living used this type of music when they were having the residents do exercise. By clapping and tapping their hand and feet, this would get the residents moving their body to the beat of the music.

B. Dance tunes of their era will bring back the past.

C. Slow tempo will be good when it comes time for you to get your loved one ready for bed.

When getting Dad ready for bed or getting him a bath I would put on slow tempo and Dad did much better. But it didn't always work as the disease advanced. Sometime Dad just didn't want to even have music on. He would say that the lowest tempo was too loud for him. So we would just turn all the music off and Dad was happy.

Please remember that after you have put your loved one to bed, please turn off the music for the evening so they can sleep. You also need to remember that each person has likes and dislikes of the type of music they enjoy.

3. *Anxiety management.* When our loved one becomes nonverbal in the later stages of Alzheimer's, he or she often becomes very uptight, and by engaging them in music activities, it can calm their mood and make them feel better about themselves. The best way we can see if music will work with our loved one is to watch them and see how they act at certain times of the day. Then you will be able to judge which music can help them to calm them down during the day.

4. *Emotional closeness.* As the disease progresses in them, they will begin to lose their ability to share thoughts and emotions with the world around them. However, they can still move to the beat of the music, until the very last stages of the disease.

Music was a way that Dad enjoyed life and music also brought back memories of his yesterday.

STORYTELLING

Creating a time to tell stories about the family is a way to bring your loved ones memory back.

Storytelling active are also being used today in adult day care, nursing homes, and assisted-living facilities. Family can also use this type of actives in their home when taking care of their loved one. Storytelling will stimulate your loved one's memory.

Let's look at how storytelling can stimulate the mind and memory.

1. It can encourage communication.
2. Promotes self-esteem.
3. Doctors say that using storytelling as an activity is a good way to stimulate the memory, imagination, and creating new memories for our loved ones.

Now let see how we can put a story time together and make it enjoyable for our loved ones.

A. *Create the right scene.* The first thing we need to do is to eliminate noise by turning off the television and radio.

   When is the best time to have your story time, in the magic hours of the day, 9:30 a.m. to 11:30 a.m. or right after lunch.

   You need to maintain eye contact when you are telling a story.

B. *Choose pictures carefully.* When using pictures don't use family pictures, because this can bring on yes and no answers. The better pictures to use are unrealistic, bright colors, animals, and pictures that bring back the past.

C. *Learn questioning,* don't ask a leading question, our loved ones will answers the question with a yes or no answers. Open-ended questions are the best to ask in storytelling.

D. *Be persistent.* When telling a story to your loved one if they do not respond to what you are saying, try to tell the story the next day, and see if they response to you better. It could take some time for your loved one to understand the story that you are telling them, but just give them time, and at the same time have other members of your family come in and have stories time with your loved one, story time can also bring your family closer together.

E. *Keep a stiff upper lip.* When our loved ones uses negative language, incorrect language, bathroom language, or sexy language, don't frown on their answers. This could make your loved ones become afraid, as well as not take part in the activity any more.

F. *Integrate music.* You can add music to your story time, music will help bring your loved ones memory back as you tell the story.

G. *Go with the flow.* Story time don't need to be written down, you can use your imagination.

H. *Redefine story.* You do not have to put a beginning, middle, or end to your story. Just go with the flow

PICTURES

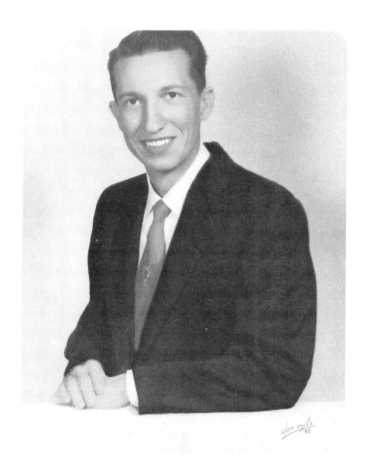

Richard Johnson as a young man

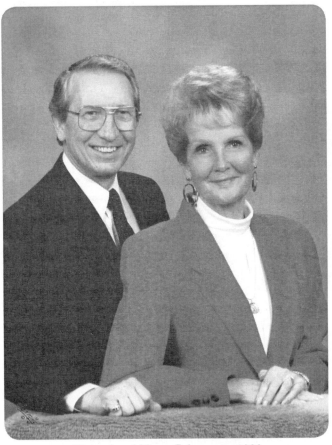

Richard and Nancy Johnson in 1992

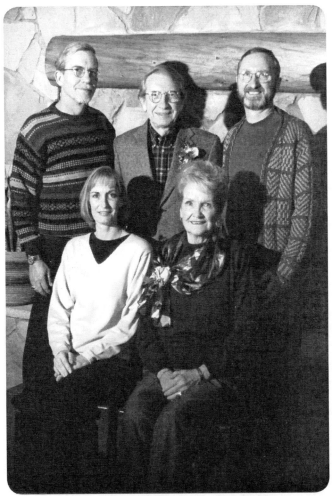

Family picture taken at Dad and Mom's, (Richard
and Nancy's) fifth wedding anniversary

PROJECTS YOU CAN MAKE WITH OR FOR YOUR LOVED ONES

One of the things that I love to do for Dad was to make memory projects. Not only did these projects help Dad with his memory, but they also taught our family about his life. One day I happened to be talking to Dad's oldest grandson, Tony, and read him the story that we had put together for Dad's story board. Tony told me that he never knew the things that the story talked about; he was so glad that we were trying to keep Dad's memory alive.

I hope that these projects will bring you and your loved one lots of fun and joy and at the same time teach your family about your loved one and where they come from.

CARE BOX

The care box plays a big role in the way that we care for our loved ones when we have to take them to the doctors, the emergency room, or on an outing. Having the care box would have made life easier for us and Dad when he had to be taken to see the doctor or go to the emergency room. The box would have also been good to have when we were moving from Indiana to Alabama. Dad just did not have the patience to wait for the doctors or when we were taking him on an outing.

This is a list of things that I put in Dad care box, when I made one for him.

1. First choose the type of container you would like to use for your loved one.

   Think of the hobbies that your loved one loves to do.

   A. We chose a fishing box to use as Dad's care box, since he loved to fish.

2. Change of clothes
   A. Night clothes
   B. Underwear or diapers
   C. Socks or slippers

3. A little first aid kit is good to have.

4. Personal needs
   A. Shaving cream
   B. Aftershave
   C. Disposable razor for men
   D. Makeup for women
   E. Deodorant
   F. Body wash
   G. Shampoo and conditioner
   H. A comb or brush
   I. Toothpaste and toothbrush
   J. Mouthwash
   K. Antibacterial wet ones
   L. Hand sanitizers are good to have on hand
   M. Gloves, for you in caring for your loved one.

5. Snacks
   A. Juice in little boxes (Please keep a look out for the date on the box that tell you when to use it by).

B. Crackers or cookies are good to keep in your box; you'll never know when your loved one will need to have a little snack.

6. Most of all, your loved one's box needs to have an object for stimulation.

This will keep their mind working and not think of how long it is taking the doctor to see them or when you will be at your destination.

MEMORY BOOK

Making Dad a memories book was one of the things that I loved to do for him. Being able to tell his story and teach his grandchildren and great-grandchildren about their grandfather was also a great way for me to get to know more about my father-in-law by finding papers, letters, and cards that told about his life.

Also looking through pictures gave us a way to look back into Dad's family. We are able to see how much Dad loved his wife, children, mother, father, and also his two brothers and sister. This also gave me the time to call family members and ask them what they knew about a family member, and this got us all taking about Dad and the family.

Scrapbooking is not hard to do; all it takes is time and lots of love. When you start to lay out the pictures and see how you want the pages to look, all of a sudden your story is coming to life.

As I worked on Dad's scrapbook, my mind came alive with his story. So enjoy the time you spend remembering your loved one. This is also a good way that grandchildren can have one on one with their grandfather or grandmother. What a great way for them to make memories that will last a life time.

MUSIC ALBUM

In making a music memory book of their favorite songs, all you need for a music memory book is a book or album that will hold CDs and the words to the songs that your loved one likes to hear. You will need to also have a little CD player that you can take with you.

Having a music album will give your family a chance to see and hear what type of music was being played when Granddad and Grandma were growing up. This can be lots of fun for the whole family to enjoy and also learn from.

STORY BOARD

A story board is also a good time to have your children learn more about their granddad or grandma; it is also a good way to bring learning and fun together for the whole family, at the same time our loved one's story board will also help the staff of the nursing home and assisted-living facility to get to know your loved one better.

These are the things that I look at when I was making Dad story board. I hope they will give you some ideas for your own story board for your loved one.

A. What their likes and dislike are.
B. Did they serve in the armed services?
C. What they did in their early years.
D. Who are the members of their family?
E. What type of hobbies they like to do?

F.   Where they went to school or college.

This is a great tool to help with your loved one's care. It will make life much easier for everyone that is involved with your loved ones care.

I can tell you that when I brought Dad's story board into Ashton Gables for the first time, Dad's caregiver, Pam, told me how much she had learned from the story board about Dad that she did not know before.

Making Dad's story board was lots of fun; we were able to take a walk back into his life. Looking through pictures, we also found his appointment papers to Annapolis, the United States Naval Academy. I talk with family members to find out if they knew anything about Dad as a young boy and asked my husband and his sister if they had anything that they wanted to add to the story about their Dad. Writing and making the story board has given me new ways to tell our family about their grandfather and great grandfather and most of all that Dad is the most loving and kind father, grandfather, great-grandfather that any family could have.

The story board, care box, and music album were given to me, from Cheryl Thrasher, the executive director of Ashton Gables; today she is the executive director of Lakeview Estates. These were some of the tools that she used when her mother was in a long-term care facility. Like all families, we all want to be able to bring back our loved one's memories. By using these tools, the family is able to take a walk back into their loved one's life. So please enjoy making these projects for your loved one.

MAKING YOUR HOME SAFE FOR YOUR LOVED ONE

Making your home into a safe place for your loved one that has Alzheimer's can reduce accidents and increase their well-being. Also, making your home safe can give you as the caregiver, peace of mind and will reduce your stress, as you care for your loved one.

I put together this checklist to help me out when I was safe proof my home for Dad and Mom when they moved in with my family. If I didn't have this list I knew that I would of miss something that I need to look into and make sure our home was safe for Dad and Mom.

1. Clean all passageways.
2. Remove unnecessary furniture, knickknacks, clutter and items that may cause confusion.
3. Fix loose, broken or uneven steps, and handrails
4. See that gates are put at top of stairways.
5. Install safety latches on cabinets that store dangerous items, such as knives, firearms, medications, and cleaning products.
6. Place guards around radiators and other heaters.
7. Install secure locks that are higher or lower than eye level on outside doors and windows.
8. Remove all poisonous houseplants.
9. Keep small objects that may be swallowed out of sight.

10. Make sure electrical wires and phone cords are secured and cannot be tripped over, and lamps that cannot fall over.
11. Remove or fasten down throw rugs to prevent slipping.
12. Put nightlights in bathrooms, hallways, and bedrooms. I need to put 25watt light bulbs all around the house, so Dad would not full at night.
13. Make sure light fixtures are easy to turn on, such as switches near doorways.
14. Use maximum wattage allowed by fixtures.
15. Reduce light glare with frosted bulbs (blue or pink).
16. Ensure adequate lighting by stairways and passageways.
17. Remove stove oven knobs when not in use.
18. Install an automatic shut-off switch on the stove.
19. Put away kitchen appliances such as blenders and toasters.
20. Use nonslip decals or mats in the tub and shower.
21. Install grab bars around the tub, shower, and toilet.
22. Try a bathtub bench or a hand-held shower.
23. Keep the temperature gauge on the hot water heater at 120 degrees or lower to prevent scalding.
24. Remove locks on bathroom doors. You never know if your loved one will lock the door, and then forget how to unlock the door.

Dad did that one day and thank goodness our lock just need to have a nail to pop it open.

But I did remove the lock, and from that day on Dad never lock himself in the bathroom.

If you have any lock on inside doors they need to be removed. I am talking also about the bedroom as well. Just remember that our loved ones will forget that they lock the door and they will not be able to get out, and they will become very frighten.

25. Outfit your loved one with an ID bracelet or some other form of identification.

26. Obtain a wristband transmitter or other tracking device to locate wanderers.

27. Post emergency telephone numbers in large print near phones, if they can still read.

I place a little piece of paper in Dad wallet, with importation phone numbers, if Dad wanderer off. But for us Dad was didn't wanderer off that much. See we made shore that everyone knew about Dad and his Alzheimer's. We lived in a neighborhood that looked out for each other. It was also great having the Sheriff live down the street from my house. So the Sheriff men always made their rounds down my street.

28. Prepare and practice an emergency exit plan.

29. Don't leave your loved one at home alone, even for a few minutes. You will never know what they can do in that time while you are gone. If you need to go out, please ask a family member or a friend to come and stay while you are out. This also goes for if you are going out in the back yard too. One day I was going out to see to

my plants and at the same time Dad headed out the front door. After about a half hour I went back in to get some water and see how everyone was doing. I ask Mom were Dad? She didn't seem to know where he had gone to. Thank God we had windows all around our house, when I look out the front windows there was Dad siting on the bench under the tree in the front yard. I went to see if he was ok, and from that time on when I went outside I made sure that Dad came with me. We made siting area under all the tree we had around the house so Dad had place to sit when he was with me, and I never lost him again.

ASKING YOUR DOCTOR QUESTIONS ABOUT ALZHEIMER'S DISEASE

These are some of the questions that I asked our family doctor.

1. Does Dad have Alzheimer's or other dementia disease?
2. Do we need to have more test done?
3. Should Dad see a specialist for his Alzheimer's?
4. What kind of treatment are you recommending will help Dad with this disease?

     These are just some of the questions that I ask Dad doctors, about his Alzheimer's...est. You might have more questions to ask your doctor. Just ask all the information that you need to take care for your loved one in the right way. The more that we know the better caregiver we can be.

THESE ARE SOME OF THE IMPORTANT THINGS THAT YOU NEED TO DO AND TAKE TO THE DOCTOR APPOINTMENTS

When Dad came to South Carolina, and after I had seen to all Dad and Mom legal and financial planes. The next step was to get them to see all their new doctors, for each of their problems. As for Dad we need to see his family doctor first so he could recommend Dad to a good Neurology that would see to his care as well as his Alzheimer's.

1. We were on time for Dad appointment.
2. Stayed with Dad thought his whole appointment.
3. I saw that the following was taking to the doctors,
   A. Our Power of Attorney (POA) for health.
   B. All Dad medications, that includes prescriptions and over the counter that Dad was taking.
   C. Before going to see the doctor, I made up a complete family heath history.
   D. I tried to give the doctor all the information that I could about Dad's health and I didn't worry what he thought because I know that what I was doing was for him because I love him very much, and the doctor was the only one that could help Dad through this disease.

EMERGENCY ROOM VISITS

You need to stay with your loved one and see to all of their needs, answer all the doctors' questions, and make sure that you have brought all of their paperwork from home that will be needed in the emergency room. I made up two folders to keep all of Dad and Mom's paperwork in and also had empty bottles of their medicine that they were taking that year, I kept this bag in my car. So when we went to the doctor, all I had to do was take the bag in with me.

When I had to take Dad to the emergency room, I made sure that he was with me at all times. When we got to the emergency room the first thing I did was to tell the attendant that Dad had Alzheimer's disease and what stage he was in. I also made it known that Dad had a hard time with waiting to see the doctor. I let the attendant know that a person with Alzheimer's/dementia disease doesn't have the ability nor the patient to wait a long time to see the doctor. I also ask if there was another room or a quiet place where Dad could wait for the doctor to see him, and explain that a person with Alzheimer's disease does not like noise, and an emergency room can be very noisy.

I always brought Dad's care box, memory book or his music album with us to help keep Dad at ease, as he waited for the doctor. Once we got into the room and the nurse started to ask me question about Dad health and his Alzheimer's, I would pull out my big bag of goodies that I always carry with me. Not only did I carry the important paperwork for my family but I also carried Dad and Mom's paperwork with me. Their Power of Attorney (POA) for health and a copy of do-not-resuscitate order or living will, as well as IDs and insurance cards, and phone numbers of family and doctors that need to be called were always with me. In my car I kept empty bottles of their medication, so when the nurse asks me what Dad was taking I just hand her the bag. I always waited until the doctor asked me any questions about Dad, as well as waiting to the end of the examination to ask the doctor any questions I might have.

All through the appointment, I kept telling Dad that I love him and was not going anywhere, till we were done with the doctor.

LIFESTYLE CHOICES

Seeing what Alzheimer's disease can do to a loved one. We need to make a big change in the way we lived. One way was by caring for our brain health. This is one of the most important things that we can do for ourselves. Here are some tips that my husband and I use to help keep our brain cells working and give us a better and healthier lifestyle.

1. You need to see the doctor, at least once a year.
2. You also need to be tested for Alzheimer's disease after the age of sixty-five.
3. You need to do activities that will stimulate your brain, like read, play memory games, work on crossword puzzles, play cards, chess, and any other games and mental exercises that will put your brain to work and not just sitting in front of the TV all the time. Some of the things that I love to do is sew for my niece, do needlepoint, read, and work in my flower garden.
4. Handle your stress by having time away, relaxation, getting a massage, having time with the Lord, meditation, and exercise is also good for the brain. Every day I have time with the Lord, work out in my flower garden for about one hour, before I start my day.
5. We need to treat depression the right away.

A. Our loved ones that have depression are at a high risk of getting Alzheimer's or other dementia in their lifetime.

B. Depression will lower your loved one's quality of life.

C. Depression also brings with it a higher rate of death among our loved ones that have Alzheimer's or dementia.

6. *Social.* You need to get out and see family and friends. This will help with the overall level of your brain stimulation.

7. We need to exercise on a daily basis. (Walk for about thirty minutes a day.)

8. Physical activity greatly reduces the chance of cardiovascular problems that could cause Alzheimer's disease in our loved ones as well as you.

9. We need to control diabetes and heart disease, which put us at a higher risk for Alzheimer's.

A. Physical exercise and not smoking keeps our blood pressure under control.

B. Lower our cholesterol.

C. Keeping our weight under control. These physical activities cannot stop the disease from happening, but we can try to keep this disease from coming into our lives.

10. We need to have a good diet and take vitamins daily. You need to take vitamins C, D, E, and B complex supplements.

11. Having a good eating habit. Eat good food like fruit, vegetable, poultry, and fish. Please keep in

mind when eating beef and pork, it should be eaten in moderation. Following and developing good eating habits will help us to stay healthy, and at the same time our brain will have a better chance also. I am not saying that this will stop us from developing Alzheimer's or dementia disease, but it can help us live a better life as we get older.

12. Alcohol has a very bad effect on our brain; and kills our brain cells as well.

STRESS MANAGEMENT

It is very important that we handle our stress, because stress can damage our body and our mind. These are some of the stress relaxation methods that we (my husband and I) use when we start to feel stress coming on.

1. *Meditation.* Emptying the mind of thoughts to aid mental or spiritual development.

2. *Guided imagery and visualization*
   A. Guided imagery is done with tapes. They suggest you to see yourself on a beach or other beautiful places.
   B. Visualization is where the person creates a mental picture of something in their mind.

3. *Deep breathing,* where a person will breathe long deep breaths that come from the bottom of the lungs to the top of the lungs and then exhaled out. This will give the person a relaxation feeling. Any breathing relaxation techniques can work

for you. Just give about twenty-five to thirty minutes every day.

4. *Classical Music.* Our ears are connected to our brain, which is connected to our central nervous system. When we listen to loud music, it sends our brain into a hostile or aggressive behavior. But when we listen to classical music, it puts our brain into a pleasant behavior. That sends us into relaxation mode.

5. *Massage.* Treatment that involves rubbing or kneading the muscles of the body. Getting a massage is a good way to give your mind a good rest, from a long stressful day or week. (Roger and I try to get a massage every now and then).

6. *Prayer.* When we have time with God and make a spiritual life for ourselves, we are able to manifest it in many ways. Stress that is given to God will bring forth a healthy life, in the following ways.

   A. We stop smoking.
   B. We stop drinking.
   C. Enhanced spirituality.
   D. Spiritual living is linked to better medical outcomes when treatment is necessary, as well as less sadness and hopelessness, and a will to live a long and happy life.
   E. While all forms of prayer are good for stress management, short prayers that are vocal will be the most useful to reduce your stress.

You do not have to do all of these relaxation methods, just whatever makes you feel better about yourself, and work a few minutes every day on one of these stress management relaxation methods. I use prayer for my relaxation every day. Having time with God put me into a very unstresful environment, and I am able to work and care for my family in a better way.

PRESCRIPTION DRUG COVERAGE

I like to give to some help on prescription drug coverage. When Dad and Mom came to live with us one of the first things that I had to do was to get them on a good insurance plan that would take care of their medication. See Dad medication would cost us about $500.00 a month, and Mom cost us about $800.00 a month. So you see that having prescription drug coverage is very importation to your loved ones.

Here is some information that I found, when I was looking for coverage for Dad and Mom. I hope it will help you and your loved one get the right coverage. "With prescription drugs on the rise, we need to have ways to pay for our loved one's medicine. As the disease of Alzheimer's worsen over time, Medicare is one of the places that we can get help from. Medicare: 1-800-633-4227 or visit www.medicare.gov.

Here are four points that can help you with Medicare Part D

1. *Eligibility.* To receive Medicare part A and B and Medicare advantage plans.
2. *Enrollment.* From November 15 to December 31 of each year.
3. *Plans.* That will best fit your loved ones needs.
   A. Brand name of your loved ones medicine
   B. Generic drug coverage

    C. Pharmacies or mail-order companies that can fill your order under the Medicare part D plan

4. *Cost*. You will have a monthly cost that is set by the insurance companies, for the plan you choose.

Other cost that you are responsible for are as follows:

A. Copayment.
B. Deductible.
C. Once you have paid your loved one's deductible, their benefits will apply to their policy. Please read your policy carefully and always ask questions of your insurance companies.

You will find other insurance companies that can help you with Medicare Part D as well. Remember to check and see if these other companies will cover hospitalization and doctor visits.

EDUCATIONAL RESOURCES

These websites are very good to get more information on how to deal with the disease of Alzheimer's or dementia:

"Alzheimer's Foundation of America
322 Eight Avenue, Seventh floor
New York, New York
Phone # 1-866-232-8484
www.alzfdn.org "[53]

STATE GOVERNMENT RESOURCES (ALABAMA)

"Alzheimer's Association
Phone # 1-800-272-3900
http://wwwalz.org"[54]

"Alzheimer's of Central Alabama
PO Box 2273
Birmingham, Alabama 35201
Phone # 205-871-7970
www.alzca.org "[55]

FEDERAL GOVERNMENT RESOURCES

"Alzheimer's Disease Education and Referral Center
PO Box 8250
Silver Spring, Maryland 20907
Phone # 1-800-438-4380

www.alzheimers.org   www.nia/nih.gov/Alzheimers/
AlzheimersInformation/GeneralInfo"[56]

"The United States Food and Drug Administration (FDA)
10903 New Hampshire Avenue
Silver Spring, MD 20993
Ph. 1-888-INFO-FDA (1-888-463-6332)
http://www.accessdata.fda.gov/scripts/cder/ndc/default.cfm
(When you are in this website, you need to do the following.)
1. National Drug Code Directory,
2. Then go over to the right and click on Proprietary name search.
3. Search by Proprietary Name: In the search box place the name of the drug you are looking for when it first came out on the market."[57]
www.cms.hhs.gov

"Department of Health and Human Services
200 Independence Avenue, SW
Washington, DC 20201
Phone # 1-877-696-6775
www.hhs.gov "[58]

"US Department of Veterans Affairs
810nVermont Avenue NW
Washington, DC 20420
Phone# 1-800-827-1000

www.va.gov"[59]

"Eldercare Locator
61 Medford Street
Somerville, Massachusetts 02143
Phone # 1-800-677-1116
www.eldercare.gov "[60]

"Employee Benefits Services Administration, US Department of Labor
Frances Perkins Building
200 Constitution Avenue, NW Room 5625
Washington, DC 20210
Phone # 866-444-EBSA (866-444-3272)
www.dol.gov/ebsa"[61]

FDA for Older Persons
5600 Fishers Lane
Rockville, Maryland 20857
Phone # 1-888-463-6332
http://www.fda.gov/oc/seniors"[62]

"USDA Food and Nutrition Service
3101 Park Center Drive
Room 926
Alexandria, Virginia 22302
Phone # 1-703-305-2052

www.fns.usda.gov "[63]

"National Institute on Aging
Building 31, Room 5C27
31 Center Drive, MSC 2292
Bethesda, Maryland 20892
www.nia,nih.gov "[64]

"US Administration of Aging
Washington, DC 20201
Phone # 1-202-619-0724
www.aoa.gov "[65]

"US Social Security Administration
6401 Security Blvd
Baltimore, Maryland 21235
Phone # 1-800-772-1213"[66]

"US Senate Special Committee on Aging
G31 Dirksen Senate Office Building
Washington, DC 20510
Phone # 1-202-224-5364
www.aging.senate.gov"[67]

"United State Census Bureau
4600 Silver Hill Road
Washington, DC 20233
Phone # Call Center: 301-763-INFO (4636) or
800-923-8282
http://www.census.gov "[68]

LONG-TERM CARE

Long-term care is assistance or supervision for a person that can no longer care for their daily needs.

"The United States Department of Health and Human Services said that seventy percent of Americans that are over the age of sixty-five will need some type of long-term care services in their life time, and twenty percent will need long-term care for more than five years.

"There are a number of factors that contribute to Americans needing long-term care.

1. *Age.* As we live longer we will need more long-term care.
2. *Marital status.* A person that is single is more likely to need the services of long-term care than a person that is married.
3. *Gender.* A female will need long-term care more than a male, because females have a longer lifespan. Females who live over the age of 65, on the average lives 3.7 years longer than a male who lives on the average of 2.2 years.
4. *Lifestyle.* The way that we live, eat, and exercise will determine our need for long-term care services.
5. Our *health.* Like, family history." [69]

This part of my book is the hardest for me to write. The day will come when our loved ones will need around-the-clock care. I would like to tell you how we came to the reality that we needed to move Dad into an assisted-living facility. In the beginning of this book, you were told that Roger had to move to Madison, Indiana, so he could take on a new job, and I would remain in South Carolina caring for his Dad and Mom till we sold our home. Where do I start to tell you how the next year would teach me to lean on God more, and how God would send my church family and friends to help me out, when our families was not around when I needed them? This also made me grow stronger in my faith as well.

After Christmas 2007, I went for a little time off from being a caregiver. We needed to prepare our family for the move to Madison, Indiana, in August; at the same time we needed to look for an assisted-living facility for Dad, when the time came for him to have round-the-clock care.

As I returned home from my trip to Madison, this is when my world would came tumbling down around me, and with God's help, I was able to get through this time. The day after coming home from Madison, I went to church to see if the Christmas decorations had been put away. Sometime in the late afternoon, I took the flowers that had wilted over Christmas to the back to be thrown away. Our pastor's wife, Lynn, came to the back of the church and started to call to me: something had happened to Benjamin, (Benjamin is my seventeen year old son, who had and accident on his high school track.) He was getting ready for soccer when he passed out. He was taking to the Medical College of Georgia

(MCG) were we would found out in the week to come that Benjamin has Epilepsy, like other members of my family.(Me, and my Uncle) and we needed to get to the school right way. When Ms. Lynn and I arrived at the school, Benjamin was on the ground, and the paramedics were working on him. All of his team mates had gone into prayer and were asking God to take care of him. One of the schoolteachers who was also a member of my church was waiting for us. She had a look on her face that you knew something was not right; she took my hand and walked me over to where the paramedics were. With God's help, I was able to keep clam. The paramedics were going to have to take Benjamin to the Medical College of Georgia (MCG). MCG was the only hospital that had a trauma unit in our area; it was also an hour's drive from Barnwell.

Our pastor let it be known that our family needed help with Dad and Mom. That night our pastor and Ms. Lynn took me to MCG; they did not want me to drive by myself. When we arrived at the hospital, I asked to see where Benjamin was. They told me that we were going to have to wait and someone will come and talk with us about his condition. As we waited to hear what was going on with Benjamin, Ken said to me, "Martha, do you think that you need to call Roger and tell him what is going on?" I then called Roger to let him know what had happened to Benjamin and let him know that I did not know how long we would be in the hospital. About midnight Ms. Lynn came and told me that she and Ken needed to head home. At the same time we still did not know what was going on and what they were going to do. We ended up staying all night, and the next day a good friend, Mama Ruth, who is like a mother to me, went over to my home to see that the caregiver had made it in for the day. Mama Ruth told the caregiver that she would be back with dinner right before she left for the day. At the same time, she sent her husband, Papa James, and Papa Doyle, with my car, cell phone, and my medicine so I could go back and forth from the hospital. Benjamin would have to stay in the hospital for a week, and I would have to spend my days between the hospital and home. By the time I placed my head down on my pillow at night, it seemed to me like I had been up for two days. God was with me the whole time. Every night as I left the hospital, my cell phone would ring, and Ms. Lynn was on the other end wanting to know where I was. Just hearing her voice made me feel better, knowing that someone cared about me. All I could think about was how was I going to make it through this time, with no family around to help me out.

Benjamin and I were not home from the hospital more than a week when we would be back in the hospital, but this time it was my mother-in-law. Dad was getting more and more impatient with me. One night about three week after Benjamin came home from the hospital. The doctor allowed him to go back to his after school job. But the law state that a person with Epilepsy can't drive for six month, that is why I was taking Benjamin to work, Dad bugged and bugged Mom about dinner. Instead of Mom telling Dad to wait until I got back from bringing Benjamin to work, she got up and went to start dinner. As she started to prepare dinner, she lifted a heavy iron skillet that caused her to crack two vertebrae in her back; by the time I got home, she was in pain and thought that she had pulled a muscle. Well, we put her to bed and watched her for about three days. On the third day, we were back in the hospital. Dad was not going to go to the hospital with me; he said hospitals are where people go to die, and he was not ready to die yet. This time Dad was going to make the trips to the hospital a lot harder for me, and at the same time, Benjamin was having test on his heart. This meant that I would have to race the clock to be at both hospitals on the same day and would have to make it home before the caregiver left at 2:30 p.m.

This is where you can say that God carried me in his arms. He even sent the good people of Hagood Baptist Church to be my guardian angels, and my big sister, Cindy, was always there for me. Cindy would be there when I needed her just to talk, cry, or laugh.

No sooner did Mom come home from the hospital than she was right back in, but this time she went in for chronic obstructive pulmonary disease (COPD), and she would not be coming home right from the hospital. She would have to have rehab for twenty-one days. It would be while Mom was in rehab that Dad would have an Alzheimer's breakdown.

One night when I was so tired and had gone to bed right after I had put him to bed, about eleven o'clock, Benjamin came home from work. He came into my room and woke me up, by saying, "Mom, Grandpa has made a mess all over the house, and I cannot find him."

Well, I flew out of bed and walked right into a mess, but the first thing that Benjamin and I needed to do was to find where Grandpa went. We looked all over the house, and all at once, something told me to look in my bathroom. That's where I found Dad. He was sitting on a pillow, on the toilet in my bathroom, and had made a mess. I had to clean him up and put him back into bed. For the rest of the night, I stayed up and cleaned.

The next day, I called his doctor and told him what had happened during the night. The doctor said that Dad was having an Alzheimer's breakdown and wanted to know what had happened that would send him into a breakdown. I told him that Mom had a COPD attack and was in the hospital, and they were going to be moving her to rehab for twenty-one days. He said that would do it! He asked me to keep an eye on Dad for a couple of days; he was also going to send some medication that would calm Dad down and help him cope. The doctor also said that I needed to talk to Roger and tell him what was going on, and we also needed to start thinking about long-term care for Dad. He told me that since he was also my doctor, he was very concerned about my health as well. The stress that Dad was putting me under was not good for my health. I called Roger and talked to him about what was going on with Dad and that the doctor was recommending that we look into long-term care for him.

When I was in Madison back in December, I had looked at some assisted-living facilities that I thought would be right for Dad when the time came. After talking with Roger, I called Hampton Oaks and asked if they had a room that was open. I told them that Dad had had an Alzheimer's breakdown, and the doctor was recommending that we look into long-term care, since we did not have family around to help me out with the twenty-four-hour duties. You can say that God was looking out for me in my time of need.

Hampton Oaks told me that a room had just come open and if I could have Roger give them a call so they could set up an appointment for him to meet with them, they could get all the paperwork done within two weeks. Roger could kill two birds with one stone: he could come home to move his dad to Hampton Oaks and tell his mom what the doctor had said. I was right back on the phone to Roger. You can say that God had his hand in seeing that all of the paperwork was done within four days. By Thursday, Roger called me to tell me that he was coming home.

This would be a turn-around trip that would make the trip to Barnwell, South Carolina, and back to Madison, Indiana, a long and hard trip for him. I would not be able to go with him; Mom needed someone to stay and see to her needs. As for Dad, the trip was no problem; all he did was doze the whole way, and this made the trip a little easier for Roger.

When Roger had finished moving Dad into Hampton Oaks, he was invited to have dinner with his Dad. At dinner, Roger asked him how he liked the trip to Madison, Indiana. Dad said, "What trip?"

That night when Roger called to tell me that they had made it safely, he told me the story of how Dad did not even know that he had gone on a trip. I knew in my heart that we had made the right decision on Dad's care. Now I had the job to tell Mom that Dad was in good hands, and it would be just a few months before we were on our way to Madison ourselves.

When Mom came home from rehab, she became a handful, and I started to see some of the warning signs in her, but I knew that her warning signs were not the same as those of Dad's. Mom's warning signs were caused by her COPD because of the lack of oxygen that was not getting to her brain. She also missed Dad very much; we had time to sit and talk about Dad and made phone calls so she could talk with him.

One night when Roger and I were talking on the phone, I told him that his mom was getting depressed, because she could not see Dad. He said, "Why don't you and Mom come to Madison, and she can see Dad all she wants for a whole week. That will make her feel better, and she will be able to cope till we move in August."

I said it was a great idea, and the next day I made plans for us to go to Madison and see Dad.

So please remember that your loved ones are still husband and wife, and this will be one of the hardest times that they will have in their life, being apart.

MAKING IT EASIER FOR OUR LOVED ONE TO TRANSITION TO RESIDENTIAL CARE SETTINGS

Making the transitioning from your home to a residential care facility, you, the caregiver, and your loved one that has Alzheimer's will have a hard time with this move. You have to understand that for many years, you have been on call twenty-four hours a day, and now you are about to come off that twenty-four-hour on-call period. Now you have to let someone else take over your role as caregiver. As for your loved one, they will have a hard time with their new surroundings. You will need to give them some time to get used to their new home and the staff that will be caring for them.

When I was looking for an assisted-living facility for Dad, these were some of the questions that were on the top of my list to ask. I would not settle for just any facility for Dad; it had to be the best we could afford.

1. *Look for a good, clean and qualify facility:* As a caregiver, when you are looking for a long- term residence you need to look for the following.

    Are they caring and loving to the residents that they care for?

    Is the dementia care unit staffed with professionals that have been trained in dementia care?

    Do they keep up to date with training for their staff?

    Do they give all the time that is needed to the family when they have questions about the facility?

    Do they walk you through the facility and tell you what they offer for care for your loved one?

    Do they sit down with you when it comes time to go over the paperwork and answer all of your questions that you might have?

How far is the facility from your home or work? Will this distance allow you to go and visit your loved one?

2. *Does the residence meet the following specifics?*

Medical. Does the residence have a medical director on staff?

Social. What types of activities and daily needs are provided to the residents?

Therapeutic. What type of treatment is given in the caring of their residents with Alzheimer's or dementia disease?

Emotional. What type of emotional care is given when they are having a bad or blue day?

3. *Understand the emotions at play.* Your loved one may give you some problems when they first move into their new home. Just keep saying to yourself that your loved one needs round-the-clock care that you can no longer give them.

You must understand that your loved one will not understand why you or your family have made this decision.

Your loved one's new surroundings may overwhelm and confuse them.

If you stay away for about four to five days, your loved one will have time to get used to their new home and time to get used to the staff.

4. *Provide input.* At the same time, you need to share what you have done and how you have cared for your loved one over the years with the following staff members.

        Executive director
        Resident services director
        Nursing staff
        Social worker
        Nutritionist

5. All of this should be done prior to admission into the facility.

    The nursing home or assisted-living facility staff needs time to get to know about your loved one:

        Medical condition
        Temperament
        Behavior patterns
        Likes and dislikes and so on

6. *Talk about it.* You need to talk to your loved one about their upcoming move into a nursing home or assisted-living facility. By talking to them about this move, it will make the move a little better for them and you.

    Telling your loved one about the move is a decision that you, the caregiver, must make.

    This should be based on your loved one's understanding of the situation.

    If your loved one has a hard time with understanding why they have to move into a nursing home or assisted-living facility, you can talk about this every day, till the day of the move.

    Let your loved one have a chance to express their concerns and fears.

    Please be patient with your loved one.

Have some understanding with your loved one.

Tell your loved one that you will come to see them weekly.

7. *Prepare their room before they move in:* This is the most important thing that you can do for your loved one when time comes for them to move into the nursing home or assisted-living facility.

If you live in the same town as the nursing home or assisted-living facility, you will be able to set up your loved one's room right away. But if you are moving from out of town or out of state, see if you can bring some things with you until the rest of your loved one's things arrive. When we had to move Dad from Madison, Indiana, to Birmingham, Alabama, while unpacking the boxes, we found the things that we would need to decorate in Dad's room, and at the same time, we wanted to make Dad's room look like a little apartment. When new pictures of his great-grandson would come out, we always bring a new one for him to see. Even though Dad cannot remember who we are, he is still a member of our family that we love very much.

So when you are setting up your loved one's room, think of what they would like and also try to put family memories in their room also.

Set up room before they move in with their furniture. We set up Dad's room with his bed, dresser, night table, and his chair that he loves.

Put family objects and pictures in their room.

Label all their clothes.

Label all personal items.

See that they have seven days' worth of cloths, towels, and two sets of sheets.

8. *Be by their side:* On the day of the move, accompany your loved one to the nursing home or assisted-living facility.

Tell them that they will be okay and that you will stay with them for the day.

Have dinner with them at the facility.

When it is time for you to go home, please tell your loved one that you will come back soon.

Let your loved one know that they will be fine and that the staff will do a good job caring for them.

9. *Introduce your loved one to the staff of the nursing home or assisted-living facility.*

Let the staff know that your loved one is new to the facility.

10. *Check in regularly.* It is still your responsibility to see to the needs of your loved one.

Show support to your loved one, with the staff of the nursing home or assisted-living facility.

11. *Think about yourself.* You need to have your family or friends to be able to comfort you at this time.

You have been the one caring for your loved one all of this time, and all at once it has come to an end.

Give yourself some time.

Seek support from others who have been through this with their loved one.

You can also talk to the staff of the facility that your loved one has moved into.

Your loved one's nursing home or assisted-living facility will host a family night once a month.

You need to remember that you are doing this for the good of your loved one and your health. So remember that God knows just how much you can do, and he knows of the love that you have for your loved one, and also remember that your loved one is in good hands.

HOW TO PLAN FOR LONG-TERM CARE

Before you or your loved one are diagnosed with Alzheimer's or other dementias, this will be the best time for you to start planning for your or your loved one's long-term care. Also, look at nursing homes or assisted-living facilities at the same time. The reason that you need to make a visit to the nursing home or the assisted-living facility is to see what they have to offer in caring for you or your loved one when time comes for round-the-clock care. Not all nursing homes and assisted-living facilities will care for Alzheimer's residents. The other reason that you are looking at nursing homes and assisted-living facilities right away is that some facilities need to put your name or your loved one's name on a waiting list; this depends on the area that you are looking into.

When Dad came to live with us in South Carolina after we had made sure that all financial and legal issues where taken care of, the next step was to look for a good nursing home or assisted-living facility, which played a big part in our planning for Dad's care and seeing that things were in order when the time came for Dad to need more help.

I would like to stop here for just a minute to talk to you about when you promise your loved one about moving them into a nursing home or assisted-living facility. Don't say that you will never put them into a nursing home or assisted-living facility. You don't know what is going to happen over time while your loved one is with you.

Roger and I told his dad and mom that we would keep them home as long as we could. There would be a day that we would not be able to care for them at home anymore. We would make sure that the nursing home or assisted-living facility that they would move into would meet our standards of living. I need to tell you that my standards were set very, very high. We were only promising what we could do, and also knew that someday we were going to need more help with Dad and even Mom before she passed away in January 2010. This was also a time that we asked God to lead us in the right direction in planning for Dad's and Mom's care.

Here are some things that you need to talk to your family about when you are planning for your loved one to move into a nursing home or assisted-living facility.

1. The whole family must come to a total understanding of this matter. If there is misunderstandings and disagreements between family members, then no one will come to have

a good understanding of all the facts that need to come out about why you need to move Dad or Mom into a nursing home or assisted-living facility. Every one needs to have a say in this matter, so each one will not feel guilty or angry about it.

One weekend when it was my brother-in-law and sister-in-law's time to come and care for Dad and Mom, we all had a talk about how we were going to care for Dad when time came for him to have round-the-clock care. Roger and I told them that we would keep Dad at home as long as we could and at the same time I was looking at nursing homes and assisted-living facilities. We were going to have to put Dad's name on their waiting list, and it could take up to about two to three years for us to get a room for him. My sister-in-law told us that we needed to put Dad and Mom into an assisted-living facility as soon as possible. I told her that Dad and Mom were Roger's, Craig's, and Carmen's parents and that God had asked all of us to care for them as they had cared for their children as they were growing up. I reminded her that in Ephesians 6:2–3 that God tells us that we need to "honor our Father and Mother." Even though we are their daughters-in-laws, this commandment still applied to us also. So as long as they are living in South Carolina and when the day came for them to move in to our home, Roger and I will honor what God has asked us to do. She also didn't like that Roger had promised his Dad that he would take care of him as long as he could, and when the day came for him to be moved into a nursing home or assisted living facility, we would move him into one of the top facilities that we could find in the area.

So that is why I am saying that you all need to come to a total understanding in this matter. You can see that not all members of your family will look at caring for your loved one in the same way as you do, and they will not have the same understanding of what your loved one would want when they have to be moved into a nursing home or assisted-living facility.

2. Why should we move Dad or Mom into nursing home or assisted-living facility?

   The reason that Roger and I had to move Dad into an assisted-living facility, was that he needed round-the-clock care, and with Roger being out of town, Mom being in a nursing home for rehab, and not having any family around to help me with Dad around-the-clock care. My doctor didn't think that I could care for Dad twenty-four hours a day and still see to the needs of my children and at the same time keep up with my health also.

3. What is the cost of caring for Dad or Mom in a nursing home or assisted-living facility, and where is the money coming from?

   Dad and Mom did a good job of saving for this part of their life. But they did not know that

Alzheimer's was going to come into their lives and eat up a lot of their income for an assisted-living facility for Dad.

Roger and I looked into how and when Dad or Mom would be eligible for Medicaid. When all of their assets had been used up, we even looked into Veterans' assistances, since Dad had served in the navy. We found out that Dad and Mom had to use up their assets to about $65,000 for both of them together and only $20,000 for Dad after Mom had passed away. This is for both assistances service (Medicaid and Veterans).

So the earlier that you plan, the better it will be for you, your family, and your loved one. These are a few of the things that Roger and I were looking at when we were planning for Dad's and Mom's care. I hope that these things will help you in your planning for you or your loved one's care.

4. See if their income will get them through this time in their life. In most cases, social security and their pensions will not cover all of the cost of long-term care.

Dad's social security and his pension only cover half of his assisted-living bill for the month. We have to go into his savings to get the rest.

5. Their assets (real property or investments).

6. Will your loved one receive help from other family members? This depends on your family.

7. Does your loved one have long-term care insurance? One of the best things you can do for yourself or your loved one is to buy long-term care insurance.

   This is the one thing that Dad did have for a little bit, but as for Mom, she stopped her long-term care insurance, thinking that she would not need to have long-term care in her lifetime. May I tell you that was one of the biggest mistakes that she made back in November 2009, when she got sick and had to be moved into an assisted-living facility. Having both Dad and Mom in an assisted-living facility, it would have helped us out a lot if Mom would have kept her long-term care insurance.

8. If your loved one has served in the Armed Services, you might be able to receive Veterans' benefits.

9. The following are things to consider when looking for a nursing home or assisted-living facilities.

   A. When you have put a list of nursing homes or assisted-living facilities together, you need to make an appointment to meet with the nursing home or assisted-living facility administrators and staff, and at the same time you would want to visit the facility.

   B. Before you go to visit the nursing home or assisted-living facilities, you need to do your homework on the facility. These are some of the websites that you can use when looking for a nursing home or assisted living facility.

1. This "website www.medicare.gov/NH Compare/home.asp"[70] is where you can search for nursing home or assisted-living facilities by state, county, city, or zip code. On this site you can view several different types of information that includes the following, facility, characteristic, inspection, staffing level, and quality information. This site will also give you a facility overview of basic characteristics of each facility. Like, type of ownership (for profit, nonprofit, church related, etc.), type of payment accepted (Medicare, Medicaid, or both), the size of the facility, and whether the facility is part of a chain. All of this information can be very helpful for you in finding a good nursing home or assisted-living facility for you or your loved one; this also can help you weed out nursing homes or assisted-living facilities that don't meet your standards.

2. See if the nursing home or assisted-living facilities that you are looking at have passed their "State Nursing Home and Assisted Living inspection. Reports can be found on their website: www. medicare.gov/NHCompare/home.

asp"[71] and click on the button labeled "Inspections."

Before visiting the nursing home or assisted-living facility, ask these following questions on the phone.

C. Do they have an opening, or how much time will it take for you to get your loved one into their facility?

D. See if the nursing home or assisted-living facility can accept the financial source that you or your loved one will be using.

E. Will the nursing home or assisted-living facility take long-term care insurance?

F. When will we need to put in for Medicaid (medical assistance from the government for people that have no other way to support themselves)?

G. When will we need to put in for Veterans' Affairs?

H. Are there any fees?

I. What is the monthly cost?

J. Does the facility meet all state standards for caring for their residents that have Alzheimer's?

10. I would like to give you some questions to ask on your first visit. If the nursing home or the assisted-living facility cannot answer yes to these questions, they might not know the answer to your questions. So please go by your feeling and keep looking for the right nursing home or the assisted-living facility that will make you and

your family feel right about placing your loved one in this facility.

A. Does the nursing home or the assisted-living facility have their license up to date with the state?

B. Does the administrator have their license up to date with the state?

C. Does the nursing home or the assisted-living facility meet all state fire codes, because it is hard to move people that have Alzheimer's or dementias out of their room when there is a fire?

D. Does the nursing home or the assisted-living facility keep up with their training of their staff monthly or yearly?

E. Does the nursing home or the assisted-living facility respond quickly to the call light?

F. If the residents can't use the call light and has to call out, does the staff respond quickly?

G. See if you can stay for meal time to see how the facility cares for their residents.

H. See if it is all right for the family to fix up their loved one's room.

I. Can the family come at any time to see their loved one? If the facility only has set visiting hours, you need to ask why you don't have the right to see what happens at all times of the day.

J. Is the staff cheerful, warm, pleasant respectful, and do they interact with the residents?

K. Does the administrator get to know the residents?

L. Does the staff enjoy working at the facility and with the residents?

M. Is the facility clean?

N. Are the residents kept well groomed, clean, well fed, and safe at all time?

O. Do the residents seem happy and love to be living in this facility?

P. Does the facility engage in daily activities with the residents?

Q. How many staff members work on each shift?

R. If you do not understand what is being said, please ask questions. This will be your loved one's new home, and you need to know every thing about the facility and how they will care for your loved one.

S. See that all financial agreements are put in writing, and you need to ask for copies of all paperwork that you signed.

T. If the staff beats around the bush in answering your questions, this should tell you how they will treat your loved one and your family after your loved one moves in to the facility. You then need to look for a better nursing home or the assisted-living facility that will meet your set standards.

U. When it comes to use Medicare or Medicaid, you need to make sure that the nursing home or the assisted-living facility is certified to take Medicare or Medicaid residents into their facility.

1. If you are paying your loved one's nursing home bills with their money and over time you will need to have assistances with Medicaid, see how long the waiting time is.

2. You need to find out if they will keep your loved one or will you have to look for a new home when your loved one goes on Medicaid.

V. Are all agreed dates of when you will move your loved one into the facility and what care will be furnished by the facility? (All of this should be written in the contract.)

W. Under what conditions will the resident be asked to leave the facility?

Will it be over?

1. The decline of their health?

2. Their behavior?

3. Problems walking?

4. Incontinence?

5. How much time will the nursing home or the assisted-living facility give you to find a new facility?

6. Does the nursing home or the assisted-living facility have another facility that your loved one can move to?

7. Please go over the entire contract that you have signed with a lawyer to make

sure that everything in the contract is on the up and up.

I hope that these questions and websites will help you to plan for your or your loved one's long-term care and how to look for a good caring nursing home or assisted-living facility.

PAYING FOR LONG-TERM CARE

In this section, we will be talking about how we are going to pay for our long-term care.

Long-term care has a large price tag that comes with care, especially when care is needs to be for an extended period of time. It is very important for us to be aware of what it is going to cost us for long-term care for us or our loved ones.

Health insurance and disability insurance don't cover the majority of long-term care services, and the government only pays a limited amount of the long-term care benefits that we will need. Our social security and pensions in most cases will not cover all of the cost of long-term care so that is why we need to look into other ways to cover the cost.

Long-term care cost varies from the number of nursing home and assisted-living facilities in your area or state where you live in. Also, the cost will vary by what type of care will be provided. Example will be as follows:

1. Will you be doing the caring at home?
2. In nursing home or assisted-living facility.
3. Adult day care.

4. Have someone come in from a home care service to help with your loved one.

The cost also depends on what type of care you will need for you or your loved one and how long of a time period the care will be needed. All of this will play a part in the cost of long-term care.

"According to a 2009 survey that was taken by MetLife Mature Market Institute, we can see that they took surveys from nursing homes, assisted-living facilities, adult day care services, and home care services to find out what the average cost for long-term care services are in the United States:

1. $198 a day for a semiprivate room in a nursing home
2. $219 a day for a private room in a nursing home
3. $ 3,131 a month for care in an assisted-living facility (this is for a one-bedroom unit)
4. $21 an hour for a home health aide
5. $19 an hour for a homemaker services
6. $67 a day for care in an adult day care center"[72]

Like I said, these are only average cost for long-term care services. The facility has the right to set their price for care by what they have to offer the family that uses their facility. If you want to see what the average cost are in your area, please look at this website: "http:// www.longtermcare.gov. And click on paying for long-term care, then go to the map, and click on the state that you want to find the average costs." [73]

There are several ways to pay for long-term care, which includes the following:

1. *Personal resources.* You can pay for long-term care from your or your loved ones personal income, savings, investments or other funds that you may have. In some cases, people have to sell their assets, like their home, stocks, or some even have to take out second mortgages to pay for their loved one's long-term care.

2. *Veterans.* If your loved one has served in the Armed Services, you might be able to receive Veterans' benefit, for their long-term care. "If you go to www.va.gov, and click on Veteran Services, and from there go to Health & Well Being, then A-Z Health Topic Finder, click on H, you will see the website for Health Care Eligibility and Enrollment, http://www.va.gov/he. But you need to remember that your loved one needs to qualify for these benefits. This is their phone number also 1-800-827-1000." [74]

3. "*Medicaid* is a two part joint program that takes place between the federal government and state government, that pay for part to all nursing home care for you or your loved one that meet certain criteria.

   "To qualify for Medicaid, you or your loved one must meet federal and state guidelines for income and assets. Medicaid also pays for some home and community based services, and as for assisted living facilities, they only help with very limited amount of assistance." [75]

   Many people pay for their long-term care out of their own income, and with the cost of long-term care being high, most of these people will spend their income and assets down to where they will become eligible for Medicaid. If you or your loved one are still married, and you or your loved one still remains at home, Medicaid will keep some of your income and assets for your wife or husband to live on. Also, in some states they have long-term care insurance partnership programs that help people out with insurance coverage that protect assets to meet Medicaid eligibility for you or your loved one.

4. *Long-term care insurance.* My father and mother-in-law brought long-term care insurance to see to their care when they were not able to care for themselves anymore. Like all insurance companies each of their customers is giving information on the insurance that they have purchase. As I was doing my research I came across the information that Dad and Mom had received. I thought this information would be good to place in the book, so you (my Readers) could have this information to help you and your family, to have a better understanding of what need to be done when a person is looking to buy lone-term care insurance.

We as a family do not know what is going to happen in ours or our loved one's future. That is why looking into long-term care insurance is important to your family. Long-term care insurance helps us with the planning for the unexpected and helps protect with the high cost of long-term care services that we will need in the future if we were to become seriously ill, badly injured or need supervision due to a cognitive impairment, like Alzheimer's or dementia disease. Long-term care insurance can help us, when we become unable to care for ourselves daily. Long-term care insurance covers the cost of services that are provided in our home, adult day care centers, assisted-living facilities, and nursing homes.

Certain conditions will determine when we will receive benefits; these benefits are subject to an assessment done by the insurance company representative. The policies that you pick will determent what type of benefits you will receive.

A. Here are some points that you can follow when considering buying long-term care insurance:

1. You should consider buying long-term care insurance if you have the following:

   a. You have significant assets and income,

   b. You want to protect some of your assets and income.

   c. You can afford to pay the premiums on your long-term care insurance without financial difficulty.

   d. You want to stay independent.

   e. You want to have the flexibility of choosing your own long-term care facility.

2. You should not buy long-term care insurance if you do not have the following:
   a. If you cannot afford the premiums.
   b. If you have limited assets.
   c. If your only source of income is your social security benefit or supplemental security income (SSI).
   d. If you often have trouble paying for utilities, food, medicine, or other necessities.
   e. If you are on Medicaid.

All applicants must meet the long-term care insurance underwriter standards to be eligible for long-term care insurance.

I like to give you some information that you need to know about long-term care insurance. You need to buy the long-term care insurance before you or your loved one is diagnosis with Alzheimer's or dementia disease. Because if you do not buy the insurance before you or your loved one is diagnosis, you will be turned down for having a preexisting medical condition.

3. The policy premiums for long-term care insurance will dependent on multiple points, including the following:
   a. Your age will be the determining factor; the older the person is, the higher you will pay in premium.
   b. Your health.

c. The features that you have in your policy.

d. If you buy an individual or group plan.

e. If you qualify for a discount (for example, if you have good health).

4. These are some of the features that you need to look for in a long-term care insurance policy

a. The annual premium.

b. You need to be eligible for a long-term care insurance policy.

c. Authorized, limitation, and benefits that will be placed on your policy.

d. Benefits that will produce certain requirements that are used to determine your eligibility for benefits, like inability to do a certain number of daily activities, you become cognitively impaired, the doctor certification that you need long-term care, and if you have been in the hospital and the doctor thinks that you need to have round-the-clock long-term care.

e. How will benefits be paid?

f. Maximum benefit amount (daily, weekly, monthly, or the life of the policy).

g. Joint benefits (total benefit that applies to all individuals that are covered under the policy).

h. Benefit period (a specific number of years or if those years are unlimited).

i. What is the waiting period (the number of days to wait until your benefits will begin)?

j. Stricter terms or elimination for preexisting conditions.

k. Premium adjustments.

l. Inflation protection. This increases the benefits each year to keep up the pace with inflation.

m. Group rates are available to Federal or US Postal Service employees or annuitants and members, retired members of the Uniformed Services or their spouses (or other qualified relatives) under the federal long-term care insurance program.

n. You need to ask about tax advantages on your policies (there are nontax qualified policies that you can see into).

o. Make sure that the company and agent are licensed in your state, and they are allowed to sell long-term care insurance in your state. The best place to check up on a company and agents is the state health insurance department in your state.

Make sure that your policy covers Alzheimer's disease as well.

I hope that this information will help you and your loved one to plan for your long-term care.

LEGAL AND FINANCIAL PLANNING

Having a husband that has a master's degree in finances, he was able to help me with this chapter. To be able to give my Readers very important information that will help them to see to their parents or in-law legal and financial affairs.

This was the first things that we took care of, when Dad and Mom move into our home. Not only was I taking care of them, I also was seen to their bills, and any financial need that came up in a single day. Let's take a look at what information this chapter has to offer us.

One of the most important things that we need to do for our loved one's that have Alzheimer's or dementia disease is to look at their financial and legal affairs. The sooner that we get this matter under control, the better our loved one's financial and legal affairs will be.

By planning in advance, our loved one can provide input into their decision making before they become incognitive; this also lets them name a family member to care for important issues that may come up as the disease progresses.

These are some issues that you need to consider when planning legal and financial needs for your loved one.

1. *You need to look at their financial resources and investment portfolios.*
   A. Bank accounts
      1. Checking account

      2. Saving account
      3. Money market account
      4. CD
  B. Investment accounts
      1. IRA
      2. Bonds
      3. Stock
      4. 401K
  C. Your retirement investment
      1. Social Security
      2. Pensions

2. *Insurance coverage.*
  A. Health
  B. Disability
  C. Life
  D. Prescription drugs
  E. Long-term care

3. *Long-term care options that your loved one will want for their care:*
  A. Do they want long-term care in their home?
  B. Do they want to move into a nursing home?
  C. Do they want to move into assisted living facilities?

4. *End-of-life wishes.* Does your loved one want to have the following done or not.
  A. Cardiopulmonary resuscitation (CPR)
  B. Artificial feeding
  C. Artificial breathing
  D. Palliative care (treatments to manage symptoms or relieve pain)
  E. Don't resuscitate

5. *You need to see to your loved one's estate* if it has been planned out, and the following documents are needed to be put in place:
   A. Will.
   B. Living will, which give end-of-life wishes.
   C. Durable Power of Attorney that appoints a family member to make legal and medical decisions on behalf of your loved one.
6. *Hospice care* when your loved one disease becomes terminally ill.
   A. At home
   B. In the hospital
   C. In a long-term care facility

This is one of the hardest things that we have to help our loved one with.

Dad and Mom were the type of people that did not like to talk to their children about their financial and legal affairs, even after their children were grown, married, and on their own.

As the disease of Alzheimer's progressed in Dad, Mom had to take over their finances and legal affairs. Lots of financial and legal mistakes were taking place. If they had only talked to their children about their financial and legal affairs, they would have not lost $12,000 in savings.

Having a son that has a master's degree in finances should have been the first person they should have called to ask about their finances. Roger could have helped them make a better decision.

I hope that this list will help you (children) to be able to open up the lines of communication with your loved ones before the disease of Alzheimer's or dementia take over their mind, and they make the same type of mistakes that my in-laws did.

Please remember, there are people that love to prey on the elderly. That is why I am asking you to keep the lines of communication open. I can tell you from our experience with Dad and Mom and their finances and legal affairs that if we had not taken over their affairs, we would have been in a big mess.

I would like to tell you a little story: One day after Dad and Mom had moved to South Carolina and into their own home, I was on my way to see them when a salesman met me in their driveway. I asked him what he was selling. He told me that he had an appointment with my mother-in-law so she could buy more life insurance. May I tell you that I stepped right in and called my husband right away and told him what was going on. Roger asked to talk with the salesman; he asked the salesman if he could come back on a day that he could be present. When the salesman got off the phone, he asked me why we had to be present, asking wasn't my mother-in-law a grown woman and could she not make her own decision. I told him that Roger's dad had Alzheimer's, and we were there to see and help out with anything that required them making a decision, and also Roger had their POA.

I would like to talk to the dads and moms for a little bit. You should trust your children as they become older and wiser with life. You also need to remember that as you grow older, you are going to need more and more help with your finances and legal affairs. Your children are there to help you out, and if you are like our family and have a child that has a degree in finances, please listen to your child. You did not send him or her to school just for the fun of it. *I know that if Dad and Mom had listened to Roger, they would have not lost $12,000.* So please let your children help you out with your affairs; they are not going to steal from you. You should know who among your children are better at keeping their finances and legal affairs in order. All they want to do is care for you in the best way possible.

THE CONCLUSION

As I bring our family story to an end, it is my hope that you have come to have a better understanding of what Alzheimer's is and how this disease will affect your family and how to prepare yourselves before this disease strikes you or a family member. Please remember that it is all right to talk about this disease with others.

Most of all you need to have Jesus Christ in your life as your Lord and Savior for you and your family to be able to survive Alzheimer's and any other dementia disease. Remember when your family and friends go home for the day, God is with you twenty four hours. He will never leave you.

Until this day our family has come to understand what and how Alzheimer's can affect the lives of our family members. We have watched what this disease has and will continue to do to our dad. Today Dad does not speak any more, he does not even remember who we are, does not like people to touch him. Dad even has a hard time seeing his food when it is placed on his plate. But with faithfulness, I try to see him every week, I see to his needs, make sure that I talk to the staff, to see how he is doing. We make sure that if Dad has to go to the hospital, one of us is there with him and see that he gets home as fast as we can get him there. To this day, Dad does not like to be in a hospital; he gets so scared that he starts to hallucinate that people are trying to harm him.

By trusting God with our lives, he will care for us, and if we should ever be diagnosed with Alzheimer's or any other dementia disease, we have prepared ourselves for whatever lies ahead.

I hope that our family story has brought you some comfort and also know that you are not the only one out there that has a loved one that can no longer remember who their family is anymore. Most of all, know that God loves you very much, and God knows what you can handle each and every day that you care for your loved one. Please try to enjoy the days that you have with your loved one, till God calls them home to be with him.

Know that Roger and I will be praying for your family and loved ones that have Alzheimer's and any other dementia diseases every day. May we all do what God has commanded us to do, that is, to "love each other as we would love ourselves" (Mark 12:31, NIV).

END NOTES

1. Alzheimer's Foundation of America, About Alzheimer's, Definition of Alzheimer's, 2010 http://www.alzfdn.org/AboutAlzheimers/definition.html, (accessed May 19, 2010).

2. Alzheimer's Disease Education and Referral Center, Definition of Alzheimer's http://www.nia.nih.gov/alzheimers, (accessed July 30, 2013).

3. Alzheimer's Foundation of America, About Alzheimer's, Diagnosis, 2010, http://www.alzfdn.org/AboutAlzheimers/diagnosis.html, (accessed May 19, 2010).

4. Alzheimer's Foundation of America, About Alzheimer's, Diagnosis, 2010, http://www.alzfdn.org/AboutAlzheimers/diagnosis.html, (accessed May 19, 2010).

5. Mayo Clinic, Definition, Huntington's disease, http://www.mayoclinic.com/health/huntingtons-disease/DS00401, (accessed March 8, 2011).

6. Mayo Clinic, Symptoms, Huntington's disease, http://www.mayoclinic.com/health/huntingtons-disease/DS00401, (accessed March 8, 2011).

7. Mayo Clinic, Causes, Huntington's disease, http://www.mayoclinic.com/health/huntingtons-disease/DS00401, (accessed March 8, 2011).

8. Mayo Clinic, Complications, Huntington's disease, http://www.mayoclinic.com/health/huntingtons-disease/DS00401, (accessed March 8, 2011).

9. Mayo Clinic, Lifestyle and home remedies, Huntington's disease, http://www.mayoclinic.com/health/huntingtons-disease/DS00401, (accessed March 8, 2011).

10. Mayo Clinic, Coping and support, Huntington's disease, http://www.mayoclinic.com/health/huntingtons-disease/DS00401, (accessed March 8, 2011).

11. Mayo Clinic, Coping and support, Huntington's disease, http://www.mayoclinic.com/health/huntingtons-disease/DS00401, (accessed March 8, 2011).

12. Mayo Clinic, Definition, Parkinson's disease, http://www.mayoclinic.com/health/parkinsons-disease/DS00295, (accessed March 8, 2011).

13. Mayo Clinic, Definition, Parkinson's disease, http://www.mayoclinic.com/health/parkinsons-disease/DS00295/, (accessed March 8, 2011).

14. Mayo Clinic, Symptoms, Parkinson's disease, http://www.mayoclinic.com/health/parkinsons-disease/DS00295/, (accessed March 8, 2011).

15. Mayo Clinic, Causes, Parkinson's disease, http://www.mayoclinic.com/health/parkinsons-disease/DS00295/, (accessed March 8, 2011).

16. Mayo Clinic, Risk factors, Parkinson's disease, http://wwwmayoclinic.com/health/parkinsons-disease/DS00295/,   (accessed March 8, 2011).

17. Mayo Clinic, Complications, Parkinson's disease, http://mayoclinic.com/health/parkinsons-disease/DS00295/, (accessed March 8, 2011).

18. Mayo Clinic, Lifestyle and home remedies, Parkinson's disease, http://www.mayoclinic.com/health/parkinsons-disease/DS00295/, (accessed March 8, 2011).

19. Mayo Clinic, Lifestyle and home remedies, Parkinson's disease, http://www.mayoclinic.com/health/parkinsons-disease/DS00295/, (accessed March 8, 2011).

20. Mayo Clinic, Coping and support, Parkinson's disease, http://www.mayoclinic.com/health/parkinsons-disease/DS00295/, (accessed March 8, 2011).

21. Mayo Clinic, Prevention, Parkinson's disease, http://www.mayoclinic.com/health/parkinsons-disease/DS00295/, (accessed March 8, 20110).

22. Mayo Clinic, Definition, Wilson's disease, http://www.mayoclinic.com/health/wilsons-disease/DS00411, (accessed March 8, 2011).

23. Mayo Clinic, Symptoms, Wilson's disease, http://www.mayoclinic.com/health/Wilsons-disease/DS00411/DSE, (accessed March 8, 2011).

24. Mayo Clinic, Causes, Wilson's disease, http://www.mayoclinic.com/health/wilsons-disease/DS00411/DSE, (accessed March 8, 2011).

25. Mayo Clinic, Complications, Wilson's disease, http://www.mayoclinic.com/health/wilsons-disease/DS00411/DSE, (accessed March 8, 2011).

26. Mayo Clinic, Lifestyle and home remedies, Wilson's disease, http://wwwmayoclinic.com/health/wilsons-disease/DS00411/DSE, (accessed March 8, 2011).

27. Mayo Clinic, Definition, Vascular dementia, http://www.mayoclinic.com/health/vascular-dementia/DS00934, (accessed March 8, 2011).

28. Mayo Clinic, Symptom, Vascular dementia, http://www.mayoclinic.com/health/vascular-dementia/DS00934/D, (accessed March 8, 2011).

29. Mayo Clinic, Symptom, Vascular dementia, http://www.mayoclinic.com/health/vascular-dementia/DS00934/D, (accessed March 8, 2011).

30. Mayo Clinic, Causes, Vascular dementia, http://www.mayoclinic.com/health/

vascular-dementia/DS00934/D,
(accessed March 8, 2011).

31. Mayo Clinic, Risk factor, Vascular
dementia, http://www.mayoclinic.com/
health/vascular-dementia/DS00934/D,
(accessed March 8, 2011).

32. Mayo Clinic, Definition, Lewy body dementia,
http://www.mayoclinic.com/health/lewy-body-
dementia/DS00795, (accessed March 8, 2011).

33. Mayo Clinic, Symptoms, Lewy body dementia,
http://www.mayoclinic.com/health/lewy-body-
dementia/DS0079, (accessed March 11, 2011).

34. E medicine health, Symptoms, Lewy
bodies, http://www.emedicinehealth.
com/dementia_with_lewy_bodies/p,
(accessed February 22, 2011).

35. Mayo Clinic, Causes, Lewy body dementia,
http://www.mayoclinic.com/health/lewy-body-
dementia/DS0079, (accessed March 11, 2011).

36. Mayo Clinic, Causes, Lewy body dementia,
http://www.mayoclinic.com/health/lewy-body-
dementia/DS0079, (accessed March 11, 2011).

37. Mayo Clinic, Risk factors, Lewy body
dementia, http://www.mayoclinic.
com/health/lewy-body-dementia/
DS0079, (accessed March 11, 2011).

38. Mayo Clinic, Complications, Lewy
body dementia, http://www.mayoclinic.

com/health/lewy-body-dementia/
DS0079, (accessed March 11, 2011).

39. Mayo Clinic, Definition, Frontotemporal
dementia, http://www.mayoclinic.
com/health/frontotemporal-dementia/
DS, (accessed March 11, 2011).

40. Mayo Clinic, Symptoms, Frontotemporal
dementia, http://www.mayoclinic.
com/health/frontotemporal-dementia/
DS, (accessed March 11, 2011).

41. Mayo Clinic, Causes, Frontotemporal,
dementia, http://www.com/health/
frontotemporal-dementia/DS,
(accessed March 11, 2011).

42. UCSF Memory and Aging Center, What
is Posterior Cortical Atrophy (PCA),
Definition, http://memory.ucsf.edu/education/
disease/pca, (accessed March 17, 2011).

43. UCSF Memory and Aging Center, Symptoms
of Posterior Cortical Atrophy (PCA),
Symptoms, http://memory.ucsf.edu/education/
disease/pca, (accessed March 17, 2011).

44. UCSF Memory and Aging Center, Symptoms
of Posterior Cortical Atrophy (PCA),
Symptomshttp://memory.ucsf.edu/education/
disease/pca, (accessed March 17, 2011).

45. UCSF Memory and Aging Center,
Progression of Posterior Cortical
Atrophy (PCA), Progression, http://

memory.ucsf.edu/education/disease/ pca, (accessed March 17, 2011).

46. Alzheimer's Foundation of American, About Alzheimer's, Life Expectancy http://www. alzfdn.org/AboutAlzheimers/lifeexpectancy. html, (accessed May 19, 2010).

47. United States Food and Drug Administration (FDA),Treatment, http://www.fda. gov/, (accessed July 31,2013).

48. United States Food and Drug Administration (FDA),Treatment, http://www.fda. gov/, (accessed July 31,2013).

49. National Institute on Aging, Statistics, http:// www.nia.nih.gov, (accessed July31, 2013).

50. United State Census Bureau, Statistics, http:// www.census.gov, (accessed July 31, 2013).

51. Alzheimer's Association "2012 Alzheimer's Disease facts and Figures, Alzheimer's & Dementia, Volume8, Issue 2 http://www.alz.org/facts_figures_2012. pdf, (accessed July 26, 2012).

52. Alzheimer's Disease Education and Referral Center, Cost, http://www.nia/nih. gov/Alzheimers/AlzheimersInformation/ GeneralInfo, (accessed August 2, 2013).

53. Alzheimer's Foundation of American, Government Programs, Federal State Government Resources, http://www.

alzfdn.org/Medicare/federalresources.
html, (accessed May 19, 2010).

54. Alzheimer's Association, Government
Programs, State Government Resources,
http://www.alz.org, (accessed August 2, 2013).

55. Alzheimer's of Central Alabama, Government
Programs, State Government Resources, http://
www.alzca.org, (accessed August 2, 2013).

56. Alzheimer's Disease Education and Referral
Center, Government Programs, Federal
Government Resources, http://www.nia.nih.
gov/alzheimers, (accessed August 2, 2013.)

57. The United States Food and Drug
Administration (FDA), Government
Programs,Federal Government Resources,
http:// www.accessdata.fda.gov/scripts/cder/
ndc/default.cfm, (accessed August 2, 2013).

58. Department of Health and Human
Services, Government Programs, Federal
Government Resources, http:// www.
hhs.gov, (accessed August 2, 2013).

59. US Department of Veterans Affairs,
Government Programs, Federal
Government Resources, http://www.
va.gov,   (accessed August 2, 2013).

60. Eldercare Locator, Government Programs,
Federal Government Resources, http:// www.
eldercare.gov, (accessed August 2, 2013).

61. Employee Benefits Services Administration, US Department of Labor, Federal Government Resources, www.dol.gov/ebsa, (accessed August 2, 2013).

62. FDA for Older Persons, Government Programs, Federal Government Resources, http://www.fda.gov/oc/seniors, (accessed August 2, 2013).

63. USDA Food and Nutrition Service, Government Programs, Federal Government Resources, http:// www.fns.usda.gov, (accessed August 2, 2013).

64. National Institute on Aging, Government Programs, Federal Government Resources, http:// www.nia.nih.gov, (accessed August 2, 2013).

65. US Administration of Aging, Government Programs, Federal Government Resources, http:// www.aoa.gov, (accessed August 2, 2013).

66. US Social Security Administration, Government Programs, Federal Government Resources, (accessed August 2, 2013).

67. US Senate Special Committee on Aging, Government Programs, Federal Government Resources, http://www.T, (accessed August 2, 2013).

68. United State Census Bureau, Government Programs, Federal Government

Resources, http:// www.census.
gov, (accessed August 2, 2013).

69. Department of Health and Human
Services, Long-Term Care, http:// www.
hhs.gov, (accessed August 2, 2013).

70. Medicare, How to Plan for Long-Term Care,
http://www.medicare.gov/NHCompare/
home.asp, (accessed August 2, 2013).

71. Medicare, How to Plan for Long-Term Care,
http://www.medicare.gov/NHCompare/
home.asp, (accessed August 2, 2013).

72. MetLife Mature Market Institute, How
to Pay for Long-Term Care https://www.
metlife.com/mmi/research/long-term-care-iq.
html#findings, (accessed August 2, 2013).

73. Medicare, How to Pay for Long-
Term Care http://www.longtermcare.
gov, (accessed August 2, 2013).

74. US Department of Veterans Affairs,
Government Programs, Federal
Government Resources, http://www.
va.gov, (accessed August 2, 2013).

75. Medicare, How to Pay for Long-
Term Care http://www.longtermcare.
gov, (accessed August 2, 2013).